Diabetes Questions And Answers

More than 400 Diabetes Frequently Asked Questions

Shunzhong Shawn Bao, M.D.

Endocrinology/Diabetes Specialist

© 2017 All Rights Reserved

Publisher's Note: The information contained herein is not intended to replace the services of a trained health professional or to be a substitute for individual medical advice. You should consult with your health care professional in regards to any matter relating to your health, and in particular, any matter that may require diagnosis or medical attention.

Uncontrolled high or low blood sugar levels are dangerous, and you need to seek immediate medical care for these conditions. If you are being treated for diabetes, any changes in your existing medications are not advised without first consulting a medical professional. Additionally, any changes in your diet and exercise practices should follow the guidelines of a medical professional who has personally examined you.

Material Connection Disclosure: The publisher of this report may have an affiliate relationship and or another material connection to the providers of goods and services mentioned in this book. If you purchase any of these items contained herein, the publisher may receive additional compensation.

First Edition 2017 (7b-p)

Diabetes Questions and Answers:
More than 400 Diabetes Frequently Asked Questions
Shunzhong Shawn Bao, M.D.
James Strand, Editor

Copyright © 2017
All Rights Reserved

Published by: Ace Health Publisher
ISBN: 9781545438282
www.drbao.info

Dedication

This book is dedicated to my patients. These are their intelligent questions, for which I am grateful. These make me think and keep moving everyday. So many have overcome the seemingly impossible and reversed their diabetes. Their stories have encouraged and inspired me to write this book. This book is for them, my patients.

This book is also dedicated to my colleagues, Dr. Richard Rapp, MD, Dr. Ganesh K.V. Nair, MD, Dr. Zulekha Hamid, MD, Dr. Allen Redding, MD, and Dr. Timothy M. Boehm, M.D. for their countless hours spent in stimulating discussion and guidance.

This book is dedicated to my best friend Barbara Winter and her unending kindness and generosity. With her patience and critiques, she made this book readable.

This book is dedicated to my editor Mr. James Strand. Without his passion for diabetes and meticulous work, this book would not be present in its existing form.

At last, I want to thank all the scientists who make the discoveries that I have not mentioned. Without your work, diabetes would still be a desperate disease. Now, because of you, the future for diabetes is so much brighter and encouraging. I believe that one day we can prevent or cure diabetes. This book is intended to spread your research and your studies.

Contents

Chapter 1: Essentials you need to know after being newly diagnosed with diabetes 1

Chapter 2: 10 questions to ask your insurance company about diabetes coverage 17

Chapter 3: 10 things to discuss with your family about diabetes 20

Chapter 4: 10 questions to ask before starting a new medication 24

Chapter 5: The basics of diabetes 27

Chapter 6: Diabetic education 44

Chapter 7: How is type 1 diabetes treated? 46

Chapter 8: How is type 2 diabetes treated? 59

Chapter 9: All about insulin 82

Chapter 10: Let's talk more about eating 99

Chapter 11: Let's talk about sweeteners 115

Chapter 12: Let's answer questions about holiday eating 119

Chapter 13: Diabetes and exercise 125

Chapter 14: Diabetes and travel 134

Chapter 15: How should I prepare for a colonoscopy or outpatient surgery? 140

Chapter 16: 10 questions about vaccinations 144

Chapter 17: Let's talk more about insulin pump failure. 146

Chapter 18: Diabetes and cholesterol 151

Chapter 19: Diabetes and gastroparesis 161

Chapter 20: Diabetic foot care 168

Chapter 21: Diabetes and sexual dysfunction 173

Chapter 22: Living with someone who has diabetes 178

Chapter 23: Questions about diabetes emergencies 183

Final Words 190

Appendix: A list of all 400+ questions in this book 192

Chapter 1: Essentials you need to know after being newly diagnosed with diabetes

Diet and exercise questions

What can I eat?

The first thing people with a new diagnosis of diabetes ask is, "What can I eat?"

I put this list together. Many of my patients like it.

Stay away from:	Recommended:
all fruit juices and soft drinks	water, green tea, black coffee, 1% milk, soy milk, almond milk
pizza, tacos, chips, pretzels, chicken nuggets	salad without dressing, tuna, turkey, chicken
processed meat sausage, hamburgers, hot dogs	real meat chicken breast, turkey breast, fish
red meat	lean cuts fish- salmon, tilapia, mackerel, shrimp
egg yolks	egg whites
potatoes	broccoli, cauliflower, peppers, green beans, kale, cabbage
white bread, pasta, noodles, white rice	whole grains, all beans

Stay away from:	Recommended:
watermelon, pineapple, grapes raisins, pawpaws, mangos	all berries-raspberries, cranberries, blackberries, blueberries, strawberries, papayas, apples, cantaloupe (some are too sweet). bananas, kiwi, plums, tangerines, cherries, figs, pomegranates (control portion sizes)
snacks-avoid if possible if sugar is not low candy, ice-cream, honey, chocolate, cookies, pizzas, chicken nuggets	raw or dry roasted nuts-peanuts, almonds, cashews, pistachios, sunflower seeds, pumpkin seeds, Sugar-free Jello, 4-ounce plain or sugar-free yogurt, mushrooms, raw veggies (celery, broccoli), tomatoes, fruit (see above)
candies, ice-cream, cake, cookies	protein bars, nut bars, cheese
pancakes, fried eggs, bacon	oatmeal, egg whites, low carb yogurt
butter	vegetable oil, olive oil
fried food	grilled, baked, broiled, boiled, steamed

The key is three lows: low carbs, low meat, and low calories in drinks.

How should I eat?

You should always eat something with fiber at every meal. Eat your food with fiber first. Eat your colorful vegetables before anything else. Eat your food slowly. Try not to eat snacks, but if your next mealtime is more than five hours away, eat a light snack. Try not to eat snacks just before bed. Drink plenty of water to keep yourself well hydrated.

What can I do for exercise?

The current recommendation is that you need to have moderate intensity aerobic exercise for 30 minutes a day, 5 days a week.

Here are seven exercise recommendations:

1. Start walking if you can. Get yourself a pedometer, or use an app on your smartphone, Apple Watch or Fitbit, and many others. The point of a step counter is to track your progress, encourage yourself, and keep yourself accountable. Your goal is 10,000 to 15,000 steps a day. Be aware that tracking miles is more accurate than steps. I recommend you walk 3-5 miles a day.
2. If you can stand, do not sit. We all sit too much, and sitting is a killer. If possible, you can buy a standing desk so you can stand and work on your computer, or get yourself a treadmill desk (yes, there is a desk with a treadmill). You can walk while working on your computer.
3. Keep moving if you can. Moving is always better than sitting.
4. Choose an activity you like. Think back to your childhood for sports you enjoyed, and pick them up again if you can. If this was a team sport, look around and ask your friends and family if there is a team you can join. You can also look on the internet for interest groups to join.
5. Always start slow and increase activity gradually, especially if you have not been active for a long time. It may take some time for you to build strength.
6. Listen to your body. Stop activity if you have severe shortness of breath, chest pain, or any pain anywhere. You may need to call your doctor to have your heart, lungs or joints evaluated.
7. Ideally, you can join a gym and get a qualified trainer. Most of the time, if you pay money, you will be incentivized to exercise more, because you'll want to get your money's worth.

How much weight should I lose?

Any weight loss is helpful. 5-10% can be your initial target. I have a patient who lost half of her body weight and was able to stop all her medications for diabetes, blood pressure and cholesterol.

A1c questions

Diabetes patients are talking about A1c. What is it?

A1c is short for HbA1c, which measures a 2-3 month average of blood sugar. We usually check it every 2-3 months. Sometimes we check it more often if a patient's blood sugar is too high and under active treatment adjustment.

	HbA1C Test Score	Average Blood Glucose Level Mg/dl (US)	mmol/L
Action Needed	14.0	380	21.1
	13.0	350	19.3
	12.0	315	17.4
	11.0	280	15.6
	10.0	250	13.7
	9.0	215	11.9
OK	8.0	180	10.0
Good	7.0	150	8.2
Excellent	6.0	115	6.3
	5.0	80	4.7
	4.0	50	2.6

What is my target A1c?

The target for different patients is different. However, for most people, an A1c below 7.0% is reasonable. I want to see you to get your A1c as close to normal as quickly as possible. This should be done without compromising your safety.

If you are young and your organs are reasonably healthy, you want to strive to get your A1c down to below 6.0%. The American Association of Clinical Endocrinologists (AACE) set a target for most patients below 6.5%.

If you have been living with diabetes for many years and have some organ failure already, it is not unreasonable to get your A1c below 8.5%.

Is the A1c goal different for those with CAD?

As we discussed, you need to get to normal as quickly and safely as possible. Luckily, we have many safe medications. Unluckily, some insurance companies do not pay for all of these medications. Everybody should strive to get his or her sugar as close to normal as soon as it can be safely reached. If you have limited means, or other reasons, you can have a different A1c target. We call it individualized medicine.

How often should I check my A1c?

It is recommended to check it every 3 months. However, if your blood sugar is very high and you are actively changing your treatment, your A1c might be checked more often. Under some special circumstances, such as pregnancy or before surgery, your A1c may also be checked more frequently.

Diabetes Questions and Answers: More than 400 Diabetes Frequently Asked Questions

Blood sugar monitoring questions

How often and when should I check my sugar?

I make these recommendations based on the treatment regimen.

Once a day schedule

No diabetes medications and just diet and exercise. We recommend checking just once a day (see schedule below) or 1-2 times a week if you are very stable.

Once a day schedule								
Date	Breakfast		Lunch		Dinner		Bed time	Comments
	Before	2 hrs after	Before	2 hrs after	Before	2 hrs after		
1/2	X							
1/3	X							
1/4		X						
1/5		X						
1/6			X					
1/7			X					
1/8				X				
1/9				X				
1/10					X			
1/11					X			
1/12						X		
1/13						X		
1/14							X	
1/15							X	
1/16	X							
1/17	X							

If you are on oral medications, except sulfonylureas (most common are glimepiride, glipizide, glyburide), or glinides (most common are Starlix, Prandin), then you also need to check once a day. You should follow the previous schedule.

Twice a day schedule

If you are on **sulfonylurea or glinides**, I recommend checking your sugar two times a day.

Twice a day schedule								
Date	Breakfast		Lunch		Dinner		Bed time	Comments
	Before	2 hrs after	Before	2 hrs after	Before	2 hrs after		
1/2	X	X						
1/3	X	X						
1/4			X	X				
1/5			X	X				
1/6					X	X		
1/7					X	X		
1/8							X	
1/9	X							
1/10							X	
1/11	x	X						
1/12	X	X						
1/13			X	X				
1/14			X	X				
1/15					X	X		

Morning and bedtime schedule

If you have basal insulin like levemir, NPH, Lantus (or Basaglar), Tresiba, or Toujeo, you need to check morning and bedtime. If your A1c is still not reaching your target, then I recommend to check after meals also. You do not have to check every meal, but alternating between meals.

Morning and bedtime schedule								
	Breakfast		Lunch		Dinner		Bedtime	Comments
	before	after	before	after	before	after		
1/2	X						X	
1/3	X						X	

Four times a day schedule

If you are taking multiple shots a day, you need to check sugar at least 4 times a day.

Four times a day schedule								
	Breakfast		Lunch		Dinner		Bedtime	Comments
	before	after	before	after	before	after		
1/2	X		X		X		X	
1/3	X		X		X		X	

If you have type 1 diabetes, check at least 4 times a day as above.

For type 1 diabetes, do additional tests under these circumstances:

- Check whenever you feel your sugar might be high or low.
- Check anytime when you do not feel well.
- Check before you drive.
- Check before and after you exercise to see how you respond to the exercise.
- Also check your urine ketones whenever you do not feel well.

Seven times a day pregnancy schedule

If you are pregnant, you need to check 7 times a day.

Seven times a day pregnancy schedule							
Date	Breakfast		Lunch		Dinner		Bed time	Comments
	Before	2 hrs after	Before	2 hrs after	Before	2 hrs after		
1/2	X	X	X	X	X	X	X	
1/3	X	X	X	X	X	X	X	
1/4	X	X	X	X	X	X	X	

Questions about glucometers

Which glucometer do you recommend?

The question of which glucometer you should use is a question of what your insurance will pay for and what you can afford. You have to use what you can get.

If money is not an issue, I would choose a meter that has many features: accurate, uses a very small amount of blood, and testing site versatility. When you test multiple times a day, after a week all of your fingers are tender and you do not want to touch anything. It is very nice if you can check from another site instead of only using fingers. It is also helpful if your glucometer can display your blood glucose data easily, and the data can be downloaded and printed easily. Some patients with special needs may need a meter with voiceover options and integration with an insulin pump. So far, I have not seen any meters that can do all of the above. At the end of the day, it all depends on what your insurance will pay, and what the most important features are that you prefer.

Which glucometer is most accurate?

Accuracy is very important. Unfortunately, insurance companies often dictate what kind of glucometer you can have.

If you have the choice, I would recommend Contour Next, or ACCU-CHEK. Studies show these are the most accurate meters. I really like the ACCU-CHEK FastClix lancing device also, because it minimizes pain.

I would like to have a talking meter. Which meters can do that?

Here are some meters that can talk:

- Advocate Redi-Code Plus Speaking Meter
- EasyMax Voice
- EasyMax Voice 2nd Generation
- Element Compact V
- Element Plus
- Embrace
- Fora D20
- Fora Premium V10
- Fora V12
- Fora V30
- Glucocard Expression
- Gmate Voice
- Prodigy AutoCode
- Prodigy Voice
- Solus Mobile
- Solus V2

When should I change my glucometer?

If any of the following three situations occur, you might want to change your glucometer.

1. Your insurance changes the coverage of strips, and it becomes too expensive for you.
2. You suspect your meter is not accurate any more.
3. Your meter is more than two years old.

How do I know if my meter is accurate or not?

You can purchase a standard solution to check your meter. You can also check your sugar before you go to a lab. Then you can compare the lab result with your own result. If the lab results are within 15% of your meter, then your meter is considered accurate. Here is an example. If your lab sugar result is 100, then your meter can report any number from 85 to 115.

I have financial difficulties. What can I do to lower my cost for strips?

Insurance companies are very powerful. They decide which meter and strips to cover and not to cover. Believe it or not, sometimes the copay price is higher than the cash price of the strips.

Here are seven companies that offer affordable strips:

- **Agamatrix.** Their meters are around $20.00 and the strips are 20-25 cents per strip. You can visit agamatrix.com.
- **CVS.** They have a meter (CVS advanced blood glucose meter) that costs $10 -$20 and the strips cost around 20 cents per strip. CVS has other meters with strips that are more expensive.
- **Dario Health**. They have meters that cost $30-40 and strips that cost around 25 cents per strip. You can visit mydario.com or call 800-895-5921
- **Ihealth Labs**. Their meters cost $15-30 and the strips cost around 25 cents each.

- **Omnis Health.** They have a few meters and they sell strips for 10-20 cents per strip. You can visit omnishealth.com or call 877-979-5454.
- **Prodigy Diabetes Care.** They have a few meters with strips that are around 10-20 cents per strip. You can visit prodigymeter.com or call 800-243-2636.
- **Wal-Mart.** Their Relion brand is affordable. The cost of the strips is 18-40 cents each. You can go to any Wal-Mart pharmacy to inquire about them. You can also visit walmart.com.

Online reviews from users can be helpful in making your choice. There are several other companies that offer meters and strips. You might check around and see what other meters and strips are available or recommended by others. Also, your insurance might only pay for certain meters and strips.

I am checking my sugar 20 times a day. Do you have any recommendations for me?

Well, I do not think you need to check 20 times a day, but I do have patients who are doing that. If you are one of these patients, you actually have options.

There are a couple of companies you can subscribe to and you can have unlimited strips. You pay a subscription fee per month.

Here are the two companies:

- **Livongo Health.** They offer a diabetic subscription program. They also have diabetic educators for support that you can call 24 hours a day, 7 days a week. The subscription fee is $75 per month and you can have unlimited strips. Your data will be uploaded online and you can share it with other people who care about your sugar readings.
- **Onedrop.** This subscription-based program provides unlimited strips and telephone support 24 hours a day, 7 days a week. Their subscription cost is $99 a month.

Shunzhong Shawn Bao, M.D.

Insulin pump and monitoring questions

I have an insulin pump. Do you have a meter which can send the sugar information to the pump directly?

This depends on what kind of insulin pump you have. The insulin pump company teams with meter manufacturers to make these products.

- Aviva Combo (Sold only with Accu-Chek Combo)
- Contour Next Link (Interacts with MiniMed 530G with Enlite and MiniMed Paradigm Real-Time Revel)
- OneTouch Ping (Sold only with OneTouch Ping)
- Personal Diabetes Manager (Sold only with OmniPod insulin pump)

Are there meters that can send my blood sugar to my phone, iPad or computer wirelessly?

Usually, if the sugar data can be sent to a smartphone, then the data can be processed to generate an electronic sugar log, pattern recognition, data storage, or displayed in a graph. The following meters can transfer data.

- Genesis Meter
- My GlucoHealth Wireless
- OneTouch Verio Sync
- Smart Gluco-Monitoring System
- ACCU-CHEK Aviva Connect

Are there meters that can be plugged into a computer via USB directly?

Some meters can be plugged into the computer and data can be downloaded, stored, analyzed, and shared with your doctor.

- ContourNext USB can do that.

When should I look into CGM (continuous glucose monitoring)?

Anybody who can afford a CGM is recommended to have one. Right now, Medicare and Medicaid do not pay for it. In my experience, Medicare and Medicaid recipients are the people who really need it, and I am sure that CGM can save Medicare and Medicaid tremendous money by reducing hospital visits. The cost of one hospital visit is equivalent to a year of CGM. Most commercial insurance pays for CGM for type 1 diabetes patients. I highly recommend CGM for every type 1 diabetes patient if they can afford the copay.

Which CGM is the best?

In the US, we currently have two CGM systems:

- Medtronic Enlite
- Dexcom G5.

I have personally tried both of them.

The Medtronic is nice because it is integrated with an insulin pump. There is a standalone device, but my understanding is that you may not be able to get the standalone device.

Dexcom G5 is the standalone device. I tried it on myself, and I like it very much. It is licensed to be worn for 7 days but I restarted it and wore it for 10 days. It was still very accurate and I did not experience any problem. The data can be viewed on an iPhone and you can share with anybody! Dexcom also teamed up with insulin pump companies and offered integrated pumps but was always one generation behind like the t:slim G4 insulin pump, Animas Vibe system.

Blood sugar, cholesterol and weight targets

What sugar target should I shoot for?

Different patients have different targets.

1. If you have not had diabetes for very long and have not experienced organ failures, I recommend the following:
   - Your blood sugar target should be as close to normal as possible.
   - Your fasting blood sugar should be as close to 100 mg/dl as possible.
   - 2 hours after the meal, your blood sugar should be below 140 or as close as possible.
2. For most patients, if you have had diabetes for a few years but have been reasonably fine without severe complications or other comorbidities, I recommend these targets:
   - Fasting blood sugar - below 140.
   - 2 hours after a meal - below 180.
3. For patients with many complications or prone to have severe hypoglycemia or low sugar unawareness, I recommend the following targets:
   - Fasting blood sugar - below 180.
   - 2 hours after meal - below 240.
4. For patients during pregnancy or those with type 1 diabetes or type 2 diabetes associated with pregnancy, your blood sugar targets should be:
   - Premeal, bedtime, and overnight - 60–99 mg/dl (3.3–5.4 mmol/l)
   - Peak postprandial glucose -100–129 mg/dl (5.4–7.1 mmol/l).
   - Your A1c target should be less than 6.0%
5. For gestational diabetes, I recommend diet and exercise first. The sugar targets are as follows:

- Preprandial (before meal) - less than or equal to 95 mg/dl (5.3 mmol/l) and either
- One-hour post meal – less than or equal to 140 mg/dl (7.8 mmol/l) or
- Two-hour post meal – less than or equal to 120 mg/dl (6.7 mmol/l)

What is my cholesterol target level?

The target for cholesterol is controversial, but I strive to get most of my patients with diabetes to get bad cholesterol (LDL) down to below 100 mg/dl.

If you have a history of one of the following conditions, your LDL target should be below 70 mg/dl or below.

- myocardial infarction (heart attack)
- angioplasty
- bypass
- stable and unstable angina
- stroke
- TIA (transient ischemic attack)
- carotid endarterectomy or carotid artery over 50% blockage
- other artery procedures-like iliofemoral stents or bypass

What should my blood pressure target be?

It is very important to control your blood pressure. Controlling your blood pressure can protect your kidneys, heart, eyes, and brain. Your blood pressure needs to be controlled under 140/90, ideally below 130/80.

Chapter 2: 10 questions to ask your insurance company about diabetes coverage

Currently, insurance companies do not allow doctors to decide many important decisions about your diabetes treatment. The first thing you need to do after you receive your diabetes diagnosis is to call your insurance company. These are the 10 questions you are going to ask.

Does my insurance policy cover diabetes self-management education?

Some diseases are doctor's diseases. Your doctor can cure you. You have a mole. You go to your doctor. He or she removes it, and it is gone. You have appendicitis. You go to your doctor; you have surgery, and you are cured.

Diabetes is a patient's disease. It depends on self-management. Therefore, diabetes self-management education is crucial, and it will most likely be covered. You need to know how many self-management visits it covers in a year, so you can take full advantage of it.

Does my insurance company sponsor any community programs for healthy lifestyle changes?

Some insurance companies pay for community exercise programs. Some also partner with local gyms or organizations to give you discounts. Inquire about these benefits, and it might help you live a healthier lifestyle.

What kind of glucometer does it cover?

Checking your sugar is a very important part of diabetes management. It can be very costly if you do not have test strips covered. Now we have at least a dozen glucometers to choose from. The insurance company usually has its choice of glucometer brands. Although I do not agree with their choice, I usually have to go along with it.

What diabetes medications are in the formulary?

Choices for diabetes medications are expanding. We have more than 10 categories of medications with different mechanisms and more than 100 medications from which to choose. Insurance companies usually make deals with pharmaceutical companies to cover certain brand name medications. They call it a "formulary." Many newer medications are brand name, and they may be expensive, but they could be very beneficial for you. If you can get your insurance company's medication formulary list, it will save a lot of money and trouble. Your doctors can choose from your formulary or get preauthorization if needed.

What cholesterol medications does it cover?

Diabetes doubles the risk for cardiovascular disease including heart attack and stroke. We manage your blood cholesterol medications aggressively. It is important to get the formulary for cholesterol medications.

Does my insurance cover ophthalmologist's (eye doctor) visits?

We recommend that you see your eye doctor once a year regardless of what kind of diabetes you have.

Does my insurance cover podiatrist's (foot doctor) visits?

Diabetic foot care is very important. We recommend that you see a podiatrist once a year.

Does my insurance cover weight loss?

Weight loss is crucial for diabetes management. However, not all insurance policies cover weight loss medications, programs, or procedures. It will be very helpful to know your weight loss options.

Does my insurance cover continuous glucose monitoring (CGM)?

If your sugar is not stable and it fluctuates, you might also want to ask if your plan covers continuous glucose monitoring. I recommend CGM to anyone who can afford it.

Does my insurance cover insulin pumps?

If you are using multiple insulin shots a day, you should inquire about the qualifications for insulin pumps. You should ask how much your insurance policy will cover.

Chapter 3: 10 things to discuss with your family about diabetes

Diabetes is not an easy condition to deal with. It is a lifelong disease, and it is not a disease that can be cured by a medication or a procedure. It takes lifelong self-management. You will need a strong support system.

When should I share my diabetes diagnosis with my family and friends?

You need to tell your family as soon as possible. Ideally, I recommend that you convene a family meeting. They may be eager to help you and want to know how they can help. They may be scared and want to know their chance of getting diabetes and how to prevent diabetes. You can share this book with them or give them their own copy.

What should I let my family know about my diet?

Diets are so crucial. If your diet is not controlled, your diabetes will never be controlled. Controlling your diet is difficult. This is why, after spending billions on medications, many cases of diabetes cannot be controlled. You need family support because their diet will probably change too. Many diets are available, but I support a plant-based diet. Please refer to chapter 10 for more details.

What should I let my family know about my drinks?

Controlling drinks is crucial to control diabetes. Some families have their favorite drinks and some of them might need to be changed. All sodas need to be reduced and eliminated from the family shopping list. Ideally, this should also include eliminating diet sodas. Fruit juices and even 100% juices are not good for diabetics. Sweet tea needs to be switched to unsweetened tea with stevia as a sweetener. See the drink section for more recommendations.

What does my family need to know about exercise?

It would be ideal if you can inspire your family to exercise with you. For example, you and your spouse could take a walk, ride bikes, or go swimming together every day. Exercising with someone is better because it helps you maintain a consistent regimen. If you are not exercising with a family member, you need to let your family know where you are exercising and how long. This is important because hyperglycemia (high blood sugar) and hypoglycemia (low blood sugar) can happen, and it is dangerous when they do.

What does my family need to know about my new routine?

You need a better routine to deal with your new exercise needs. Your diabetes will be better controlled if you can have a consistent routine instead of living a chaotic life. In this new routine, you will take time to check your sugar every day, and keep a nice log. Checking your sugar is like looking at the road and the surroundings when you are driving. This will help you know where you are, how fast you are going, and where you are going. You will need to eat regularly scheduled meals. If you are taking medications like sulfonylureas, you cannot miss your meals. Again, exercise is recommended every day.

What does my family need to know about diabetes medications?

Medications need to be taken as prescribed, but they do have side effects. You need to let your family know what you are taking for diabetes, as well as the possible side effects, so you all can be vigilant. Your family can also help you maintain your medication schedule. I have encountered many cases when a diabetes patient was admitted to a hospital unconscious, and none of the family members knew what the patient was taking for diabetes. When your family is familiar with your medications, they can help you achieve better quality care in the hospital should an emergency arise.

How do my family and I know if I have low blood sugar?

If you are on medications that can cause low blood sugar, you need to discuss with your family the warning signs. They need to know how to help you when you are in such a situation. Most patients have weakness, hunger, blurry vision, tremors, palpitations, irritability and sweating and if severe enough, a patient can pass out. Some patients can have mood changes and others behave weirdly or have slurred speech.

Should I teach my family members how to check my sugar?

I think it is a good idea to tell them where you store all the diabetic supplies. On occasion, you might not be able to check your sugar, and if your family is not able to know if you have low sugar or high sugar, they cannot treat you. If they know where your glucometer and test strips are, they can measure your sugar and treat you accordingly.

How should I handle glucagon shots?

If you have a glucagon shot for low sugar use, you will need to let your family know where it is kept, when to use one and how to use it. This can only be used when you are not able to eat or drink anything to raise your sugar. Give the shot first and then call 911 as soon as possible. If you have an expired one, practice on it but without actually injecting yourself. You and your family can watch YouTube instructional videos together. I watched a few of them, and their technique is correct.

Do I need to tell my family about A1c and what my A1c target is?

You should tell them what your A1c target is and how you are planning to reach your target. Your family can be an important support system to help you stay on track. They can help you discipline yourself, encourage you, and cheer you on. So, tell them your A1c and how you plan to reduce it.

Chapter 4: 10 questions to ask before starting a new medication

Let's say your doctor is telling you that you need to start a new medication for your diabetes. Here are the 10 things you need to know about a new medication. You are ultimately responsible for your actions.

What is the necessity of starting a new medication?

All medications have side effects. You need to weigh the benefits and risks of the medication and compare them against your other options.

Does it have a generic version?

Money is very important to most people. If a medication is very expensive, you are not going to take it. Some drugs are available in generic versions. The brand name and generic version may be different, but most likely they are both acceptable. The FDA has rules to ensure generic drugs work. The prices can be significantly cheaper for generic drugs.

How will it help my diabetes?

You need to know how the drug works. If you know, you will have better control of your diabetes. For example, I like the medication acarbose. It blocks the digestion of carbs. When you know how the drug works, you know if you just eat salads or proteins, you do not need to take acarbose. Acarbose will have no effect on the absorption of proteins and fiber. You will understand why you need to take acarbose with your first bite of carbs and you will understand the side effects better. For example, many people cannot tolerate this medication because of too much gas. The gas comes from undigested carbs that are being fermented by bacteria in the gut. If the carb intake can be reduced, the gas problem will be reduced. If you understand how the drug works, you can understand the nuances of how you should use it and the causes of its side effects.

Does it have interactions with other medications I am taking?

Patients are taking too many medications these days, and medication interactions are becoming a major issue. I have seen many cases of drug to drug interactions causing major harm to patients. I always check for drug interactions, but doctors are too busy prescribing medications and sometimes they forget to check for interactions. This is why you need to take charge and ask about it.

What side effects do I need to watch for?

As I said, all medications have side effects. You need to know what you need to pay attention to. I have seen many cases of patients developing side effects, seeing another doctor, and the other doctor prescribes a medication to treat the side effect. It turned out that doctor is treating the side effect of one medication with another medication.

When should I stop or adjust the dose?

All medications have potential side effects. It is important to know the potential side effects and contraindications. For example, if your renal (kidney) function is failing, or you are going to have a CT scan or cardiac catheterization, metformin needs to be stopped. If experiencing hypoglycemia, insulin or sulfonylurea needs to be stopped, or the dose needs to be adjusted. Some medications are associated with certain thyroid cancers. You need to know the conditions for stopping the medication.

Should I take my medications before a meal, with a meal, or after a meal, or at bedtime?

Different medications have different requirements for when to take it. This is very important to know.

Can I double my dose if my sugar is too high?

If your sugar is too high, you need to make an appointment to come back to your doctor's office soon. It is not a good idea to double your dose. If you are on insulin, most likely you are on a sliding scale (now called correction scale), so you can follow the scale to get your sugar down. For type 1 diabetes, you need to worry about diabetic ketoacidosis (DKA). For type 2 diabetes, your medication may need to be adjusted if you have an infection, too much stress, or in rare cases, a heart attack. Therefore, if your sugar is too high, go to the ER, or call your doctor's office at once.

Can I continue my medication if I am going to have a CT scan or cardiac catheterization?

As mentioned, if you are taking metformin, it needs to be stopped. You can resume it 48 hours later if there are no other contraindications. All other medications metabolized in the kidneys need to be used cautiously.

What should I do if I am going to have a procedure like a colonoscopy or surgery?

Some medications you can continue and some need to be stopped. Ask your physician beforehand, so when the day comes you will not panic. Your gastroenterologist or your surgeon are good resources to ask. They are probably already familiar with the medications you are taking. However, the challenge is that there are always new medications, new brand names and generic names. In total, we have more than 150 actively used diabetic medications. Your gastroenterologist or surgeon may have never heard of a medication that you are taking for diabetes. So be sure to ask your endocrinologist for advice beforehand.

Chapter 5: The basics of diabetes

Questions about diabetes prevention

Can diabetes be prevented?

The answer is yes.

How can I prevent diabetes?

Type 1 diabetes cannot be prevented now, but maybe in the future. For type 2 diabetes, lifestyle modifications should be considered. Diet, exercise, and weight loss have been shown to be effective for diabetes prevention.

Diet: plant based diet; Mediterranean diet, DASH diet (DASH stands for Dietary Approaches to Stop Hypertension).

Exercise: 30 minutes of moderate intensity exercise daily.

Weight loss: 5-10% weight loss.

Sometimes medications like metformin and acarbose have also been recommended to prevent diabetes.

Does weight loss reduce my risk of developing diabetes from prediabetes?

The Diabetes Prevention Program reported 16% risk reduction with 1 kg (2.2 lbs.) of weight loss in pre-diabetes and a BMI>=24 kg/m2 (>=22 for Asians).

Does lifestyle modification and metformin reduce my risk of developing diabetes?

The Diabetes Prevention Program reported that metformin alone can reduce diabetes risk by 31%, and the combination of intensive lifestyle changes and metformin can reduce the risk by 58%.

Can rosiglitazone or pioglitazone be used for diabetes prevention?

I do not recommend these agents for diabetes prevention. These agents are called thiazolidinediones. They are controversial and there is conflicting evidence about their risks and benefits. Some potential risks can be severe such as heart failure, fluid retention, weight gain, possible MI (heart attack), bladder cancer, and osteoporosis.

Is acarbose effective for diabetes prevention?

Acarbose is called an alpha-glycosidase inhibitor which blocks the digestion of carbohydrates. In a STOP-NIDDM trial, 100 mg of acarbose three times a day reduced the diabetes risk by 25%. However, this agent can generate severe nausea and gas which is intolerable for many people.

Can Xenical/Alli prevent diabetes?

Xenical/Alli are brand names for orlistat, which is a lipase inhibitor. It blocks the digestion of fat by 30%. A four-year randomized weight loss trial revealed a 30% diabetes risk reduction.

Can estrogen prevent diabetes?

Estrogen might have an effect on diabetes development. However, the use of estrogen is very complex and you should not use any form of estrogen for diabetes prevention.

Does vitamin D prevent diabetes?

Some research suggests that vitamin D supplements may slow the development of diabetes. Although there is no concrete evidence that vitamin D can prevent diabetes, adequate vitamin D is beneficial for muscle strength and preventing osteoporosis.

Can cinnamon prevent diabetes?

The research is conflicting. However, there are no major side effects for eating cinnamon. If you believe it can prevent diabetes, it is okay for you to take it.

Does stopping smoking prevent diabetes?

Smoking has been suggested to increase the risk for diabetes, but smoking cessation has not been proved to reduce the risk of diabetes. However, smoking cessation is recommended for everybody because the health benefits are numerous.

Can bariatric surgery prevent diabetes?

Obese patients can reduce their risk of diabetes with bariatric surgery.

Can bariatric surgery cure type 2 diabetes?

A long-term study revealed 60-80% of patients with bariatric surgery can reach long-term diabetes remission if the weight loss from bariatric surgery is sustained.

Is it true the "Little Blue Pill" Viagra can prevent diabetes?

Yes, it has been reported that the "Little Blue Pill" Viagra (sildenafil) increases insulin sensitivity, therefore reducing insulin doses for patients on insulin treatment, slowing the development of diabetes. However, this is in the very early stages of study. Viagra is not yet recommended for diabetes treatment or prevention, and you should not take Viagra for diabetes prevention or treatment.

Does more or less sleep prevent diabetes?

Quality of sleep is very important. Research has demonstrated that insufficient sleep is associated with changes in hormone secretion like insulin and cortisol. Insufficient sleep also increases the "hungry hormones" and decreases the "satiety hormones", which cause you to eat significantly more. Researchers have suggested that adults require 7-9 hours of quality sleep. The time for going to sleep is also important, and 9-10 pm is the best time to go to bed.

Can CPAP (breathing machine) reduce diabetes?

Obstructive sleep apnea (OSA) is associated with type 2 diabetes. It is estimated that 40-50% of patients with obstructive sleep apnea have diabetes already. Untreated obstructive sleep apnea causes a range of hormone imbalances like increased cortisol levels, which causes insulin resistance. The use of CPAP is the best treatment for OSA currently. Currently, there have been no clinical trials about CPAP reducing the risk for diabetes, but I think there will be. So, if you have OSA, try your best to use your CPAP.

Diabetes screening questions

Who should be screened for diabetes?

1. Significant family history– many family members have diabetes.
2. Women who have given birth to a baby more than 9 pounds or with gestational diabetes.
3. History of prediabetes.
4. Overweight (BMI>25 kg/m2) and habitual inactivity.
5. African-Americans, Hispanic-Americans, Native Americans
6. Hypertension
7. HDL<35 or triglycerides >250
8. Polycystic ovarian syndrome (PCOS)

I usually do a screening every year for patients with two or more of the above risk factors.

How do we screen for diabetes?

I usually check fasting blood sugar and A1c. In some cases, I order an OGTT (oral glucose tolerance test).

How do we do the OGTT?

75g Oral Glucose Tolerance Test

1. The patient should have no acute illnesses and not be on any diabetic medications like metformin.
2. The patient should maintain an adequate carbohydrate intake (> 150g) for at least three days prior to the test. You need to eat and drink as you usually do. You cannot be on a diet or exercise more than normal.
3. The patient should fast overnight for a minimum of 10 hours (only water is permitted).
4. 75 g oral glucose is dissolved in 250 to 300 ml of water. The patient drinks it in no more than 5 minutes. This is followed by another 100 ml of water.
5. The patient should be sitting or lying down and not move around too much. The patient should be allowed to go to the bathroom.
6. Venous blood is taken before (zero minutes) and 120 minutes after consumption of the glucose drink.
7. Urine may also be tested for glucose to estimate the renal threshold, but this does not contribute to the diagnosis of diabetes. The diagnosis of diabetes is based on the fasting and two-hour blood glucose results.

Questions about the different types of diabetes

What is diabetes?

Strictly speaking, diabetes is really not a diagnosis. It is a sign. Diabetes used to mean sugar was present in the urine, but now we understand that sugar is too high in the blood. Many reasons can cause high sugar, therefore, there are many types of diabetes.

What is insulin resistance?

It simply means that insulin is not working as efficiently as it should be. Insulin is the hormone that allows sugar to enter cells and tissues such as fat cells or muscle cells where it is metabolized. Many conditions can cause insulin resistance, such as stress, being overweight, or taking some medications.

What is prediabetes?

Blood sugar is not normal but it does not reach the diagnosis of diabetes yet. Specifically,

- fasting sugar between 100-125 mg/dl
- oral glucose testing, 2-hour sugar between 140-199
- HbA1c is between 5.7%-6.4%.

People with prediabetes can develop complications also.

What is type 1 diabetes?

Type 1 diabetes is the autoimmune destruction of pancreatic beta cells causing insufficient insulin. Generally speaking, if the patient has type 1 diabetes, insulin is required, otherwise, the patient will die. Not all diabetes treated with insulin is type 1 diabetes. For patients who developed diabetes before they were 19 years old, two-thirds of them are type 1 diabetics. Clinically, you can consider any diabetes which is prone to develop DKA (diabetic ketoacidosis) or has a history of DKA as type 1 diabetes. This is really what matters when we are talking about type 1 or type 2 diabetes.

What is type 2 diabetes?

Type 2 diabetes is the most common type of diabetes. About 90% of diabetes in adults is type 2 diabetes, while 30% of diabetes in children is type 2 diabetes. Blood sugar is high because the body cannot use insulin properly, which is called insulin resistance. At the early stages, the pancreas increases insulin secretion to make up for insulin insensitivity for the high blood sugar, but later the pancreas can fail too, which makes the diabetes worse.

What is type 3 diabetes?

Type 3 diabetes is a title that has been proposed for Alzheimer's disease which results from resistance to insulin in the brain. This has not been a broadly accepted concept yet. People who have insulin resistance, in particular, those with type 2 diabetes, have an estimated 50% to 65% risk of suffering from Alzheimer's disease.

What is type 1.5 diabetes?

In the late 1990's, some researchers coined the term "Type 1.5 diabetes," because it had features of the two major types of diabetes. They have both autoimmune destruction of pancreatic beta islet cells and insulin resistance. These patients are adults who at the beginning were more like type 2 diabetes because they could be treated with diet, exercise, and oral medications. They also have type 1 features with autoimmune destruction of the pancreatic beta cells. They also have autoimmune antibodies like the GAD antibody. Later, most of these patients need insulin. We also call them "latent autoimmune diabetes of adults" (LADA). Due to the destruction of beta cells, most of them need insulin later. Now, most doctors classify them as type 1 diabetes.

What is LADA?

"Latent autoimmune diabetes of adults(LADA) is also referred to as type 1.5 diabetes. These patients have autoimmune antibodies like GAD antibody, which indicates that their immune system is attacking their pancreatic beta islet cells. Later most patients need insulin. In the clinic, LADA is treated the same as type 1 diabetes. Patients with LADA are more stable because they do not easily develop diabetic ketoacidosis (DKA) and severe hypoglycemia.

What is gestational diabetes?

Pregnant women who have never had diabetes before but who have high blood sugar levels during pregnancy are said to have gestational diabetes. People who have gestational diabetes will have a higher risk for developing diabetes after their pregnancies. Pregnant patients with diabetes before they get pregnant are called Diabetes in Pregnancy. Both of these types of diabetes need to be well managed.

Can children have type 2 diabetes?

Yes, 20-30% of new onset of diabetes in patients younger than 20 years old are type 2 diabetes. The prevalence of childhood obesity and inactivity are expected to continue, so the childhood type 2 diabetes is expected to increase.

Can adults have type 1 diabetes?

Yes, adults can develop type 1 diabetes too. Most commonly, this is in the form of the type 1.5 diabetes, LADA, which is technically type 1 diabetes.

Are there any other types of diabetes?

Technically speaking, the diagnosis of diabetes is not even a diagnosis. It is just a symptom or sign, which means high sugar in the urine (now blood). Many conditions can cause high sugar in the urine and blood. Therefore, there are many types of diabetes. However, for most people, type 1 diabetes, type 2 diabetes, or gestational diabetes are the diagnoses.

What is steroid induced diabetes?

Since the 1940s, steroids have been increasingly used in treating many autoimmune and non-autoimmune diseases. Steroid-induced diabetes is an abnormal increase in blood sugar associated with the use of glucocorticoids in a patient without a prior history of diabetes mellitus.

What is "brown diabetes"?

There is a hereditary single gene disease called hemochromatosis. It causes increased iron absorption and deposition in organs like the pancreas and liver, which causes organ damage, and thus diabetes. The iron deposited in the skin causes it to look brown.

Early diagnosis of hemochromatosis is very important. Your doctor uses blood cell counts, iron tests, and sometime gene tests to make the diagnosis. Therapeutic phlebotomy is the treatment for hemochromatosis.

Questions about other causes of diabetes

Do night shifts cause diabetes?

Night shift worker has been suggested to increase the risk for diabetes. However, this risk has not been quantified. If you work night shifts, you need to pay more attention to your diet, exercise, and weight control.

Do sugary drinks really cause diabetes?

Based on a recent publication, 17 studies involving 38,000 people who developed diabetes over 10 years were analyzed for sugary drink consumption. It concluded that 8 ounces of sugary drinks per day increased the risk of developing diabetes by 13%. (British Medical Journal (BMJ) published online July 21, 2015).

Do plastic products cause diabetes?

There is not a concrete yes or no answer. Many products like disposable water bottles, plastic-based food packaging, microwaveable products are high in BPA (Bisphenol A) which has been shown to be EDCs (endocrine disruption chemicals), which have been linked to diabetes, obesity, thyroid cancer and other hormone related cancers.

Questions about diagnosing diabetes

How do doctors tell if I have type 1 or type 2 diabetes?

Sometimes, it can be difficult even for doctors to tell if a patient has type 1 or type 2 diabetes. Usually, type 2 diabetes occurs in overweight adults and insulin is not necessary to treat it. On the other hand, type 1 diabetes usually occurs in childhood. It usually has very severe symptoms like weight loss, severe thirst, and frequent urination. Doctors also check c-peptide and antibodies, and other blood tests that may distinguish between type 1and type 2 diabetes.

What are the symptoms of diabetes?

For type 2 diabetes, the most common symptoms are no symptoms. Therefore, blood tests are important if you suspect that you have diabetes.

Some symptoms are:

- excessive thirst
- excessive urination
- weight loss (type 1)
- weight gain (type 2)
- blurry vision
- tingling, pain, or numbness in the hands and feet

Why does my doctor say I have diabetes, but I do not have any symptoms?

The most common symptoms of diabetes are no symptoms. The diagnosis of diabetes is made by blood tests.

How is diabetes diagnosed?

A diabetes diagnosis is made by blood tests, although it is semi-arbitrary. We have four ways to make the diagnosis:

1. Fasting sugar 126 mg/dl or greater twice

2. At any time the sugar 200 mg/dl or greater and you have some sort of diabetes symptoms
3. Oral sugar testing-OGTT, 2-hour sugar is 200 mg/dl or greater
4. HbA1c 6.5% or greater

Questions about the risk of diabetes

If my brother or sister has type 1 diabetes, what are the chances for me to have type 1 diabetes?

If you have a sibling who has type 1 diabetes, the chance for you to develop type 1 diabetes is 10%. In other words, if you have one son or daughter that has type 1 diabetes, the chance of having another child with type 1 diabetes is 10%.

If my twin brother or sister has type 1 diabetes, what is the chance for me to have type 1 diabetes?

If you have an identical twin who developed type 1 diabetes, the chance for you to develop type 1 diabetes is 50%. If you have a non-identical twin who developed type 1 diabetes, the risk for you as a sibling is around 10%.

If a parent has type 1 diabetes, what is the risk for a child to develop type 1 diabetes?

If the father has type 1 diabetes, the risk is about 10% that his child will develop type 1 diabetes — the same as the risk to a sibling of an affected child. However, if the mother has type 1 diabetes, the risk for her child to develop type 1 diabetes is slightly lower, around 4%.

If you developed type 1 diabetes before age 11, your child's risk of developing type 1 diabetes is somewhat higher than these figures and lower if you were diagnosed after your 11th birthday.

Is race/ethnicity a risk factor for developing diabetes?

Type 1 diabetes is much more common in the white population. Usually, type 1 diabetes accounts for 5-10% of all diabetes in a population.

These are the most current statistics for type 2 diabetes:

- 7.6% of non-Hispanic whites
- 9.0% of Asian Americans
- 12.8% of Hispanics
- 13.2% of non-Hispanic blacks
- 15.9% of Native Americans or Alaskan Natives

Asians are a diverse group too. The breakdown of Asian Americans with diabetes is as follows:

- 4.4% of Chinese
- 11.3% of Filipinos
- 13.0 of Asian Indians
- 8.8% of other Asian Americans

My sibling was diagnosed with type 2 diabetes. What is my chance to get it?

Generally speaking, if your sibling has diabetes, it does not significantly increase your risk of developing diabetes. The exact risk is not known yet. However, if your sibling is not obese and has diabetes, then your risk is about twice the general population risk.

If my parent has type 2 diabetes and my sibling also develops diabetes, what is my risk?

If one of your parents has type 2 diabetes and one of your siblings has type 2 diabetes, your risk of developing type 2 diabetes is almost three times the general population risk. If you are Hispanic, your risk is 38.4%; if you are a black, your risk 39.6%; if you are a non-Hispanic white, your risk is 22.8%.

If both my parents have type 2 diabetes and one of my siblings developed diabetes, what are my odds of developing diabetes?

If both parents and a sibling have type 2 diabetes then the other sibling has a fourfold risk. If you are Hispanic or Black, your risk is around 50%. If you are non-Hispanic white, your risk is around 30%.

My spouse developed type 2 diabetes. Is my risk increased?

Although your spouse is not genetically related to you, you share many lifestyle habits. Depending on how similar you are and how long you have been living together, your risk can double.

Questions about doctors and doctor's visits

What are some questions I should ask my doctor about diabetes treatment?

You can ask your doctor any of the questions in this book. For every visit, you need to prepare yourself. You need to know your A, B, C, D, E and Fs.

A stands for A1c. This gauges your 2-3 months' average sugar level. Different patients have different targets. You need to ask your doctor what your target A1c is and if you have reached your target. If not, ask what the plan is to get you to your target.

B stands for blood pressure. Controlling your blood pressure is as equally important as your blood sugar. If blood pressure not controlled, it will damage your heart and kidneys, and can also cause strokes. Different patients need different blood pressure targets. You need to ask your doctor what your blood pressure target should be.

C stands for cholesterol. Controlling your cholesterol is very important in controlling your cardiovascular disease risk. Cholesterol has "good" cholesterol (HDL) and "bad" cholesterol (LDL). Again, different patients have different targets. You need to discuss with your doctor what your target should be. If you have not reached your target, ask your doctor about the plan to reach your target.

D stands for drugs (medications). You need to know what medications you are taking for diabetes, blood pressure, cholesterol, heart conditions, and for your kidneys. For your diabetes medication, you need to know how it works and the potential side effects. You also need to be clear about, any medication changes and why you need them. For more diabetes medication-related questions, please refer to the diabetes medication section in this book.

E stands for eyes and emotions. You need to have a dilated eye exam every year by an ophthalmologist and report back to your diabetes doctor, so your doctor can make appropriate recommendations for your exercise and medications. E also stands for emotions. Living with diabetes is not easy. It is common to have negative thoughts, anxiety, and depression. These negative emotions affect your diabetes directly and indirectly. You need to talk to your diabetes doctor about this, and he or she might be able to help you. Sometimes you might be referred to a specialized professional for more help.

F stands for your foot health. Diabetic foot problems can be serious. You need to report any issues to your doctor. It is also recommended that you see a podiatrist once a year.

What do I do if I don't like my current doctor?

For whatever reason, if you do not like your doctor, you should change your doctor. It is your right. Diabetes is a chronic disease. You need to have a positive relationship with your treating doctor. This positive relationship will have a positive influence on your diabetes control. Although I have not seen any research specifically on diabetes control and patient and doctor relationships, all relationships are the same. When you have a positive view of the other party, you are more inclined to accept his or her advice. Taking care of diabetes is not just about taking medications.

Diabetes care is very comprehensive. Every doctor visit should be a time to improve your self-care skills.

Are there any doctors that specialize in diabetes care?

There are so-called diabetologists who are endocrinologists who further specialize in diabetes care. The reality is that most general endocrinologist's patients are about 80% diabetes patients. Since diabetes patients frequently have other hormonal issues or endocrine problems that need to be taken care of, I recommend a general endocrinologist as your physician to help you care for your diabetes. Again, diabetes care is comprehensive care. You need a doctor who is at the forefront of cholesterol management, blood pressure management, understanding emotions, depressions, thyroid diseases and parathyroid disease. A general endocrinologist understands all these areas.

For a man, diabetes is also associated with hypogonadism and sexual dysfunction. Your diabetes doctor should be comfortable to treat that too. For women, polycystic ovarian syndrome has significantly increased risk for diabetes. Menopausal syndrome and osteoporosis are very common in women with diabetes. UTI (urinary tract infections) and dyspareunia (pain while having sex) are also common in women. Your diabetes doctor should be able to treat all these problems as well.

It would be absurd to see a doctor for every single disease. Many other endocrine diseases can also cause diabetes like Cushing's disease and acromegaly. I had a patient who was referred to me for diabetes. It turned out he had another endocrine disease which caused his diabetes.

As I discussed before, strictly speaking, diabetes is not a diagnosis. It is just a sign of high sugar in the blood.

Therefore, you will be well taken care of if you choose a general endocrinologist instead of a specialized diabetologist. In my view, a general endocrinologist is better than a doctor who just takes care of "diabetes."

How do I choose a good diabetes doctor?

There is no sure way to choose a good diabetes doctor you will like. Doctors are human too. They have different personalities. They might have certain traits you may not like, but other people might love these traits. Here are a few general recommendations when you choose a diabetes doctor.

1. Talk to your diabetic friends to ask about their experiences with a particular doctor.
2. Your PCP (primary care provider) could be a good source for information, too. Most insurance requires your PCP to refer you to a specialist. A PCP usually has experience with different specialists, and they have feedback from different patients that they use in making referrals.
3. Diabetes research and diabetes care is a fast evolving field. There are lots of new developments. You certainly want your physician, the one who treats you for diabetes, to keep up with new developments.
4. Practicing medicine is like any other profession. It is not just reading books and regurgitating what you learned. Your doctor needs to practice evidence-based medicine. Your doctor needs to apply individualization; otherwise, a machine would be able to do a better job. You need to choose a doctor who knows how to apply guidelines and recommendations to a personalized regimen that is based on your personal situation.
5. I recommend you see someone who has some professional publication experience. It is not easy to publish in a professional peer-reviewed journal. It requires a lot of research, thinking, reasoning, reading, and writing. The process of writing for a professional journal is good evidence that the doctor is really taking his profession seriously.

6. For diabetes, I think the doctor needs to be proficient in nutrition which is so important. He or she needs to be able to probe into your current diet in a nonthreatening way, then make feasible recommendations for nutritional diet changes.

7. Diabetes is such a demanding disease. It is very common for you to have negative emotions. You need someone who can cheer you up, someone who can give you an emotional lift when you are down. You need someone who encourages you when you make progress.

8. You need someone who understands general endocrinology. Since diabetes patients tend to have other endocrine diseases, you want to see a doctor experienced with other endocrine diseases. As I have said before, it would be absurd, very expensive and time consuming if you see a different one for diabetes, thyroid, obesity, blood pressure, cholesterol, and on and on.

9. I would strongly recommend a doctor who really understands cholesterol. Cholesterol metabolism is very complicated and its medications have many interactions with other medications.

10. You need to have good feelings about the doctor you choose. Just like in any other relationship, to really know if he or she is right for you, you have to try him or her. Remember, it is okay to change your doctor.

Chapter 6: Diabetic education

When should I get diabetic education?

Diabetes is a very complicated disease. It is not a single standalone disease. It affects every part and every system in your body. New treatments and new ideas are popping up all the time. We are learning and studying to keep up with it every day.

Diabetic education is ongoing. Diabetes is a lifelong disease and you need to learn every day. New situations or conditions may pop up in your life. I recommend ongoing long-term learning.

Furthermore, diabetes is a self-management disease. You have to learn every aspect of your disease and manage it. Diet, exercise, daily activity, sick days, vacation days, pregnancy, postpartum, breastfeeding, new medications and so on.

What can I learn from diabetic education?

There are many components to diabetes, such as: What is diabetes? What is the diabetes disease process? There are other aspects of diabetes you need to know about like complications, nutritional management, cooking tips, physical activity, medications and their adverse effects, glucose monitoring and psychosocial adjustment.

What do I need to do to prepare for one-on-one diabetes education?

Even if you have newly diagnosed diabetes, the chances are high that you have some knowledge of diabetes. However, this does not mean you do not need more education.

Again, diabetes is an everyday challenge. Each day may bring a new situation. I recommend you write these things down as soon as possible. Describe what happened, what you did, and the result of your actions.

Take these notes with you to your meeting with your diabetes educator. You can ask for a second opinion about what to do if this situation comes up again. Ask him or her if they have any more suggestions. Talking about specific situations like this can help your learning be more fruitful.

Sometimes, it is also okay to go to a diabetic educator and let them take the lead and listen to what they can offer.

The more you know, the more skill you will have to deal with daily challenges.

Chapter 7: How is type 1 diabetes treated?

Questions about curing type 1 diabetes

Can we cure type 1 diabetes with a pancreas transplant?

Progress is being made every day. Successful pancreatic transplants can eliminate the need for insulin injections. Unfortunately, these patients need to take immunosuppressants long-term, and sometimes they can have severe side effects. Pancreas transplants are also limited by the availability of donor organs. For now, pancreas transplants are limited to those with severe hypoglycemia with renal failure. Such patients receive pancreas and kidney double transplants.

Where can I get an islet transplant or a beta cell transplant?

There are some successful and promising cases for islet transplant or beta cell transplant, but they are still in the research stage. They are not widely available to patients yet. In America, there is a research consortium-CIT.

The Clinical Islet Transplantation (CIT) Consortium is a network of clinical centers and a data coordinating center established in 2004 to conduct studies of islet transplantation in patients with type 1 diabetes.

If you have a strong interest in transplants, you can contact the Consortium members for further information.

http://www.citisletstudy.org/

The network includes the following centers:

University of Miami Miami, Florida	University of Pennsylvania Philadelphia, Pennsylvania
Northwestern University Chicago, Illinois	University of California San Francisco, California

University of Wisconsin
Madison Wisconsin

University Hospital Rikshospitalet
Oslo, Norway

Massachusetts General Hospital
Boston, Massachusetts

University of Minnesota
Minneapolis, Minnesota

Emory University
Atlanta, Georgia

University of Alberta
Edmonton, Alberta, Canada

University of Illinois at Chicago
Chicago, Illinois

Uppsala University
Uppsala, Sweden

Karolinska University
Stockholm, Sweden

How far away is the artificial pancreas?

The artificial pancreas is an insulin pump which incorporates the continuous glucose monitor with or without glucagon to control blood sugar without the patient's constant monitoring and intervention.

This new technology is very promising and developing very fast. It will be here soon. The FDA has already cleared the Medtronic MINIMED 670G system which will be the first artificial pancreas available to general type 1 patients. The system is not yet perfect. For now, I think you should take good care of yourself and patiently wait for it to make more progress. Take care of yourself now, so when it is ready, your organs will not already be in failure.

Questions about medications, insulin pumps and monitoring

Are there oral medications for type 1 diabetes?

So far, the FDA has not approved any oral diabetic medications for type 1 diabetes. Some oral medications are off label and used with insulin, but they can be dangerous. You should not use them without a physician closely monitoring their use. There are no oral medications that can replace insulin.

Are insulin pumps better than multiple daily injections?

An insulin pump is a small computer which can be programed to deliver the insulin more precisely. If used properly, it can better control a patient's diabetes. However, usage of insulin pumps requires a degree of technological savvy. Since it is a computer, like all other computers, it can fail which can lead to very severe complications like DKA (diabetes ketoacidosis).

I recommend an insulin pump to every type 1 diabetes patient if they can afford it and are able to operate it.

Which insulin pump is the best?

Currently, there are five insulin pumps actively marketed in the United States.

Based on my experience using four of the five insulin pumps, they all are technically sound. You need to make your own decision about which one you like. Most companies allow you to try them for a month to see if you like it or not.

Here are a few things you should consider when choosing an insulin pump:

1. The first consideration should be finances. Make sure you can afford the copay for not only the initial cost of the pump, but also for supplies long term. If the copay for supplies is too high, you cannot afford the insulin pump.
2. Do you want a pump with tubing or without tubing? If you strongly dislike tubing or you have a job which prevents you from having tubing, the Insulet OmniPod is your only choice. In my experience, the cost of supplies can be high and the pod failure rate is high.

3. Do you need a Continuous Glucose Monitoring (CGM)? Can you afford CGM? Yes, you need one if you have frequent hypoglycemia. You especially need one if you have hypoglycemia unawareness. There are several to choose from:
    1) You may consider the Medtronic Pump (Medtronic 530 G with Enlite) that comes with integrated Enlite CGM system;
    2) The FDA has recently approved the Minimed 670G System, which is world's first hybrid closed loop system. If you want a closed loop system, Medtronic is your only choice for now. The Minimed 670G system is coming out in Mid 2017.
    3) Animas Vibe can display the CGM data from Dexcom G4 CGM, but it uses older-generation Dexcom data algorithm. OneTouch Vibe™ Plus Insulin Pump earned FDA approval and Health Canada License in December 2016 and is the first pump integrated with the Dexcom G5® mobile continuous glucose monitor. In my clinic, I do not have any patients on it yet.
    4) Do you want a high-tech look with a touch-screen? Tandem T slim is a good choice.
    5) Roch Accu-check Combo, which I have never used.

How can I motivate my child to check his or her sugar?

It is very challenging to motivate a child to check his or her sugar. One interesting study recently published stated that paying a child to check his or her sugar is very effective. In this study, a child can earn 10 cents to check their sugar each time, increasing daily testing from an average of 1.8 to 4.9 tests per day, with 9 out of 10 kids averaging at least four tests per day. A1c also dropped from 9.3 to 8.4 (*Diabetes Care* July 22, 2015). This study shows that incentives can be put in place to motivate children to check their sugar.

Questions about high and low blood sugar levels

Why does my sugar increase after exercising?

While exercising, stress hormones like growth hormone, cortisol, and adrenaline are released which can increase your sugar. Therefore, for some people, blood sugar can increase during exercise and 30-60 minutes after exercise, but eventually, they will come down. There are no adverse effects of temporarily raising your sugar. However, exercising is not advised if you are sick. The rise in sugar is usually more pronounced in type 1 diabetes. Therefore, we usually recommend monitoring your sugar 30 minutes after you start exercising and again 30 minutes after you finish exercising.

Why does my sugar decrease after exercising?

For most diabetics, their sugar will drop while exercising, which can sometimes last a few hours after they stop exercising. Certainly, this also depends on how strenuous and how long the exercise, and how much you eat before exercising.

What symptoms or signs might indicate low sugar?

When sugar is low, your adrenaline is secreted. It causes you to have heart palpitations, sweating, pale skin, shakiness, anxiety, irritability, tingling, anxiety, irritability, and hunger.

You might wake up drenched in perspiration and/or crying out during sleep.

As hypoglycemia worsens, you might develop confusion, abnormal behavior or both. You may also experience the inability to concentrate, and difficulty in completing routine tasks. Visual disturbances may occur such as blurred vision. If these are severe enough, they can cause seizures, loss of consciousness, or death.

What should I do if I feel my sugar is low?

You should stop whatever you are doing especially if you are driving. You also need to check your sugar and treat yourself.

How should I treat low sugar?

Usually, it is recommended you have 15 grams of carbs and wait for 15 minutes to make sure your sugar is back to normal.

Here are some examples:

- 3 glucose tablets
- one-half cup (4 ounces or 118 ml) of fruit juice
- one regular, non-diet soda
- 5 hard candies
- one tablespoon (tbsp.), or 15 ml of sugar - plain or dissolved in water
- 1 tbsp. (15 ml) of honey.

If your sugar is not back up over 70, you need to repeat the process.

I recommend that you always have some glucose tablets in your purse or in your car's glove compartment.

Depending on the situation, there are lots of other ways to treat your low sugar. If your sugar is low just before your meal, you can just go ahead and have your meal. Depending on your sugar level, and diabetes regimen, you need to adjust your medications.

What should I do if my sugar is low and I do not feel it?

Here, we assume that you do not have any hypoglycemic signs or symptoms, but your meter shows that you have sugar below 60-70. Here are two scenarios.

Scenario 1: Your sugar is not actually low, but your sugar meter is showing that it is low. In other words, the meter you are using may not be accurate. Occasionally, glucometers can have problems with accuracy.

Based on new FDA regulations, if a patient's blood sugar is below 75, the reading should be within plus or minus 15 of the actual sugar, 95% of the time. For example, if your actual blood sugar is at 70, the meter is acceptable within the new FDA guidelines to show 60.

In these situations, you need to make a judgment call. If your sugar is below 60, but close to 60, and if you are feeling fine, and if you are going to eat, you can continue your current regimen.

If you are on a multiple daily insulin shot regimen, you can give half of your premeal insulin before the meal and give the other half of your insulin when you eat or after you eat.

Scenario 2: If you have hypoglycemia unawareness, then you need to be more cautious. You have to treat every low sugar reading as an actual low sugar condition.

What should I do if I cannot feel when my sugar is low?

This is called hypoglycemia unawareness, which is very serious and has severe consequences.

Here are the five recommendations I usually give to my patients who have hypoglycemia unawareness.

1. Ask for CGM (continuous glucose monitoring) if your insurance will pay and/or you can afford it. This device can be a lifesaver for patients with hypoglycemia unawareness. For details, please see CGM section.
2. Check your sugar more often, especially before you drive (ideally not driving if possible); check your sugar before and after exercise in addition to before meals and at bedtime.
3. Use an insulin pump that will shut down if your sugar is low.
4. Talk to your doctor and he or she will raise your sugar levels, and in most cases, your sense of hypoglycemia will return.
5. Create a higher diabetes control target.

My morning sugar is always high. What can I do?

There are a few reasons to have high morning sugar.

The most common reasons are that you might eat too much at dinner or that you might eat too late at night. If this is the case, certainly, I recommend that you cut down your night meal portions and move your dinnertime earlier. Ideally, it would be good if you can take a walk after your dinner.

The second most common reason is that you might eat a bedtime snack. It is not a good idea to have a bedtime snack. I do not know who first started this idea. Bedtime snacks are the cause for weight gain. Certainly, if your sugar is low, you need to have a snack; otherwise, you do not need to eat. If your sugar consistently goes low during the night or morning, your regimen needs to be adjusted.

The third reason could be caused by the "dawn effect." This is more common in teenagers. In the morning, hormones like cortisol and growth hormones are secreted to prepare you for the morning, and these hormones increase your sugar. If this is the case, your doctor will adjust your regimen accordingly.

The fourth and most important cause, is the Somogyi effect. This effect happens when low sugar is followed by rebound high sugar. If your night sugar goes low, then your body will secrete stress hormones like cortisol, growth hormone, and adrenaline to raise your blood sugar. It can overshoot and cause your blood sugar to be high. This is actually not so common in my experience, but it is important to recognize when it happens.

As you can see, if your sugar is too low already, and if your insulin increases, then your sugar will go still lower. However, if you do not have hypoglycemia unawareness, if your sugar is too low, you will wake up sweating, with tremors, clammy, and a rapid heartbeat. If the Somogyi effect is suspected, I usually ask my patients to check their sugar at bedtime, midnight, 2 a.m., 4 a.m. and 6-8 a.m. If midnight or early morning low sugar is confirmed, then you are said to have the "Somogyi effect." You need to discuss this with your doctor and have your regimen adjusted.

The last cause is that your long-acting insulin may not be long enough. You might need to discuss this with your treating doctor to see if a change in your insulin regimen is necessary. Your doctor may increase your night time insulin, or change it to different long-acting insulin, or change it to 2 times daily, especially if you are taking Levemir.

When should I use the glucagon shot my doctor prescribed for me?

This is not for you to use. This is for family members or other bystanders to use to treat your low sugar if you become unconscious and you are not able to eat or drink. Do not use it if your sugar is simply low.

How should I use the glucagon shot?

Educate your family or whoever may be able to help you in emergency situations. Here are three recommendations:

1. After you fill the prescription, open it to review with your family or the people who might be available to help you.
2. Watch a YouTube instructional video together about how to use it and when to use it.
3. If one of your kits has expired, do not throw it away. You can use this kit to practice. Do not inject yourself; inject into a sponge or something safe.

Here are two things to remember about glucagon shots.

1. The injection sites are the same sites as insulin injection sites, like the abdomen, outer shoulder, and outer thigh.
2. Turn the patient to his left or right side since glucagon may cause vomiting.

If you have an episode of losing consciousness and you used your glucagon shot, you need to go to ER to be evaluated. They will make sure your sugar is stable and get it back up if necessary. After this, you need to visit your doctor's office to see if your regimen needs to be adjusted.

When do I need to check urine sugar?

We do not recommend checking urine sugar anymore.

Questions about ketones, high sugar and diabetic ketoacidosis (DKA)

When do I need to check urine ketones?

Ketones are produced when your body does not have enough insulin to use glucose as fuel, so it instead uses your fat stores as fuel. If severe enough, it can cause ketoacidosis which can be life threatening.

Ketoacidosis usually occurs in type 1 diabetes, although it can sometimes occur in type 2 diabetes.

However, in clinic, we usually do not discuss ketones if you have type 2 diabetes and have never had ketoacidosis before.

Under the following conditions, or any time you think you might have ketoacidosis, please check your urine ketones. You can buy test strips from your local pharmacy without a prescription, although you can also ask your doctor for a prescription.

- You feel sick, especially with nausea, vomiting, or abdominal pain.
- You cannot get your sugar under control, if you have type 1 diabetes and your sugar are persistently higher than 250.
- If you have fever, >100º F
- If your skin is flushed
- If your breath smells "fruity"
- If you feel like your thinking is "foggy"

What do I need to do if my ketones are positive?

You need to call your doctor.

Most likely, you will need to go to ER to make sure you are properly treated, especially if your sugar cannot be controlled. You may have severe dehydration.

What should I do if I have nausea and vomiting and I am unable to keep anything down?

Many reasons can cause nausea and vomiting. If this is the first time in a long time, you need to go to the emergency room or call your doctor immediately, because you may be developing ketoacidosis. This is when you need to check your urine ketones.

If you have recurrent nausea and vomiting, you may have gastroparesis.

What should I do if my sugar goes above 500 after a steroid shot?

Steroids are commonly used for many conditions, and they can increase your sugar significantly. It is not uncommon for your sugar to go over 500 after a steroid shot.

Here are the things you can do:

First, you need to make sure you do not have any other sicknesses, such as a cough or a urinary problem. If you feel really badly, go to the ER.

Otherwise, you can try the following:

- Call your doctor or visit your doctor's office for advice.
- Drink plenty of water.
- Cut down on all the carbs you are eating.
- Eat only green vegetables.
- If you are taking insulin already, increase your pre-meal insulin by 20-30% at first and then up to double your dose, and then continue sliding scale (corrections).
- If you cannot get it down, go to the ER or your doctor's office.

What should I do if my sugar goes over 500 and I am not taking steroids?

Do not panic. Calm down and ask yourself if there was anything you ate or did that may have caused the sugar spike. Try to identify the cause and see if the cause can be corrected. If you are fine and your sugar is high, you can try to correct the cause and use the sliding scale to see if you can get the sugar down.

If you have sugar over 500, and you have fever, chest pain, nausea and vomiting, or severe weakness or even confusion, you need to go to the ER.

What are the common reasons for sugar to go over 500?

Based on my patients' reports, the following 10 reasons are common:

1. Steroid use.
2. Common colds, with cold medications. Some antibiotics can cause sugar to spike.
3. Forgetting to take insulin.
4. Eating or drinking something really sweet. Something with lots of carbs even if it claimed to have" no sugar."
5. Some kind of infection, such as a UTI (urinary tract infection).
6. Alcohol- worse if alcohol is mixed with sugar.
7. Insulin pump problems (insertion cannula kinked, or inserted into a scar).
8. Expired insulin.
9. Dehydration.
10. Stress.

What should I do if for no reason my sugar goes over 500?

You need to call your doctor immediately or go to the ER.

Diabetics can have silent heart attacks which can cause your sugar to go over 500.

What should I do if my sugar is persistently higher than 250 and I do not feel well?

If you have ketone strips, check your ketones to see if you are developing DKA (diabetic ketoacidosis). If you are, go to the ER.

Please drink plenty of water to keep yourself well hydrated.

If you are on insulin, you can increase your pre-meal insulin by 20-30%, and up to 100% if needed, and continue the sliding scale for corrections. Certainly, you need to closely monitor your blood sugar.

If you are not able to get your sugar down, and if you still have chest pain or shortness of breath, see your doctor immediately. This may indicate a more serious condition, such as a heart attack.

Chapter 8: How is type 2 diabetes treated?

What is metformin?

Metformin is a biguanide that was first synthesized in 1929 and then clinically developed in the late 1950s by the French physician Jean Sterne, who gave it its first trade name, Glucophage ("glucose eater"). It was introduced as a diabetes medication in 1957 in France and in 1995 in the United States.

The discovery of metformin can be traced back to the pioneering work with extracts of the herb Galega officinalis, which led to the characterization of the blood sugar lowering effects of an active ingredient named galegine. Now metformin is synthesized.

Galega officinalis (also known by many other names including as goat's rue, false indigo, professor-weed, French lilac, Spanish sanfoin and Italian fitch) is a summer-flowering perennial herb with white, blue or purple flowers found in most temperate regions. It originated in southern Europe and western Asia, but in the last two centuries, it has spread to many countries around the globe.

Why is metformin so popular?

Here are five reasons why I believe it is so popular.

1. Metformin works. It can reduce A1c up to 1.5%. It can be combined with many other oral medications and insulin, or non-insulin injections.
2. Metformin was found to have a decreased risk of the aggregate diabetes-related macrovascular and microvascular complications and all-cause mortality in large clinical studies like the United Kingdom Prospective Diabetes Study (UKPDS).
3. Some observational data suggest that the use of metformin decreases the incidence of cancer.

4. Metformin is relatively safe, and it has been in use since 1950 in Europe.
5. Metformin is very affordable now. You can get it from many pharmacies for $4 dollars a month or $10 for a three months' supply.

Is it true that metformin might have a brain benefit?

Metformin has many positive results. Recent studies in type 2 patients also showed that those taking metformin for 2-4 years had a 40% lower risk of developing Alzheimer's disease, Parkinson's disease, and other brain and nervous system problems, while those taking the medication for longer than 4 years had an 80% lower risk.

What are the brand names for metformin?

Brands: Glumetza, Glucophage, Riomet, and Fortamet

I cannot take the big pill. What can I do?

There are two options for now. You can crush the immediate release form, or take the liquid formula. The liquid formula is Riomet.

The extended formula should not be crushed.

I cannot tolerate the regular metformin. What options do I have?

Many patients have gastrointestinal side effects, like anorexia, nausea, abdominal discomfort, constipation or diarrhea. Most patients have loose stool, or soft bowel movements, but constipation is also reported by my patients.

I recommend patients take metformin in the middle of the meal. I also recommend my patients to increase the dose slowly. Usually, I recommend my patients start with 500 mg at dinner. After a week, if tolerated, then add another 500 mg at breakfast. If your maximum daily dose is 2,000 mg after one week, increase the dinner dose to 1,000 mg, and then increase the breakfast dose to 1,000 mg.

Some patients experience a metallic taste in their mouth which can be annoying.

Extended release metformin (metformin ER) is available as generic. You can ask your doctor to switch you to generic metformin ER to try. As a matter of fact, I routinely start with metformin ER.

If your insurance pays, you can also try Glumetza which is the brand name for extended release metformin. Some patients report this is tolerated better.

I swear I saw a big pill in my stool? Has this happened with other people?

I have many patients report they have seen a pill in their stool. I have asked them to bring me the pill, but nobody has done that yet. I have never had a patient who used the immediate formula to report such an incidence. The reports came from using the extended formula, especially the brand name Glumetza.

This is actually a "ghost pill". After the contents of the pill have been released, the shell still remains. So, do not worry. Your medication has already had its effect.

Does metformin cause vitamin B12 deficiency?

Vitamin B12 is essential for nerve integrity. Vitamin B12 deficiency can cause many conditions like neuropathy, dementia, anemia and so on.

Metformin reduces intestinal absorption of vitamin B12 in up to 30% of patients and lowers serum vitamin B12 levels.

I usually check my patients' vitamin B12 periodically to make sure they are not deficient.

A daily multivitamin is also recommended.

Does metformin cause renal failure?

There is no evidence that metformin causes renal failure, but in renal failure patients, I recommend reducing the dose or not using it at all.

Does metformin cause heart failure?

It is still controversial. Some studies suggest that metformin is linked to heart failure.

I still use metformin on my patients with stable heart failure. I ask them to stop it if any sign of worsening heart failure occurs, like increased shortness of breath, cough, leg swelling, increasing dose of water pills, fever, or any sign of infection.

Does metformin cause lactic acidosis?

Metformin can cause lactic acidosis. The symptoms are nonspecific and may include anorexia, nausea, vomiting, abdominal pain, lethargy, hyperventilation, and hypotension. The mortality rate is 50%. The good news is that it is very rare if the medication is used appropriately. I have never had a patient who developed lactic acidosis.

When should I temporarily stop metformin?

You should not take metformin if you experience any of the following conditions:

1. You are very sick, with fever, dehydration, especially you have marginal kidney function or history of heart failure;
2. You are not able to drink water or have severe nausea or vomiting;
3. You are going to have a CT scan with contrast, you need to stop and I recommend at least for 2-3 days. If you know that your kidney function is marginal, I recommend you check your kidney function and then restart it.
4. You develop acute kidney failure, you should stop.
5. You develop liver failure, you should stop.

What is the best medication for type 2 diabetes?

There is no best medication; there is only the most appropriate medication. Your doctor and you should make the decision together.

Which oral medication is prone to cause hypoglycemia?

As we know, the sulfonylureas, and glinides will cause hypoglycemia. The glinides are nateglinide (Starlix) and repaglinide (Prandin).

Why are sulfonylureas not so popular now?

Sulfonylureas are not so popular now because the sulfonylureas work by stimulating the pancreas to release more insulin and are only effective when there is some pancreatic beta-cell activity still present.

The most commonly used sulfonylureas are:

- glimepiride (brand name: Amaryl)
- glipizide (brand names: Glucotrol, Glucotrol XL)
- glyburide (brand names: DiaBeta, Glynase PresTab, Micronase).

Hypoglycemia is the most common adverse effect. Sulfonylureas stimulate the pancreas to secrete insulin no matter if the sugar is high or low. It is sugar independent. It can be very dangerous in patients with kidney and liver dysfunction and the elderly.

They also cause weight gain.

Furthermore, the long-term effect on cardiovascular outcomes or mortalities is not known and may be adverse.

Why did my doctor switch me from glyburide to glimepiride?

Sulfonylureas are still commonly used in the United States for their initial effectiveness and affordability. However, in general, sulfonylureas have a high risk for causing low sugar. In particular, the commonly used glyburide is two to three times more likely to cause low sugar in comparison to other sulfonylureas used in the United States. Glyburide increases the effect of hepatic insulin sensitivity through high affinity for the cells sulfonylurea receptor, accumulation of active metabolites, and general accumulation in the islet-cell, which causes insulin release even after the medication is stopped.

Should I stop taking sulfonylureas?

You have to make the decision with your doctor. If you have taken this medication for a long time (5-10 years), the odds are very high that the medication is not working anyway. If you have other choices, you should stop taking sulfonylureas.

Do sulfonylureas cause more heart attacks?

Since 1970, The University Group Diabetes Program has raised this concern about using sulfonylureas. A large clinical trial, UK Prospective Diabetes Study (UKPDS), was initiated to address the question of sulfonylureas causing more heart attacks. The answer was NO. But ever since this conclusion, it still remains controversial. In other words, this has not been settled. In a recent analysis, it was suggested that not all sulfonylureas are the same. Relatively speaking, glimepiride is less risky and the medication of choice. It is the most commonly used sulfonylurea in the United States.

If you want to learn more about this issue, please check out this review. (Simpson, Lee et al. Mortality risk among sulfonylureas: a systematic review and network meta-analysis. Lancet Diabetes Endocrinol 2015;3:43-51)

What are DPP-4 inhibitors?

A group of gut hormones was found to be very important in glucose control. They control blood glucose through several mechanisms, including enhancement of glucose-dependent insulin secretion, slowing gastric emptying, and reduction of postprandial glucagon and reduction of food intake.

One of these important gut hormones is GLP-1 (glucagon-like peptide-1). Unfortunately, it is very unstable. The half-life is a few seconds. It turns out GLP-1 is degraded by an enzyme called DPP-4 (dipeptidyl peptidase 4). The group of medication DPP-4 inhibitors inhibits the DPP-4 enzyme, thereby increasing the group of gut hormones like GLP-1.

What are the DDP-4 inhibitors currently on the market?

Current FDA approved DDP-4 inhibitors	
Name	Active ingredient(s)
Januvia	sitagliptin
Janumet	sitagliptin and metformin
Janumet XR	sitagliptin and metformin extended release
Onglyza	saxagliptin
Kombiglyze XR	saxagliptin and metformin extended release
Tradjenta	linagliptin
Glyxambi	linagliptin and empagliflozin
Jentadueto	linagliptin and metformin
Nesina	alogliptin
Kazano	alogliptin and metformin
Oseni	alogliptin and pioglitazone
Galvus	vildagliptin (I have never used it)

Which DPP-4 inhibitor is the best?

Januvia has been on the market the longest. It is the first agent I go to. There are some possible adverse associations with some other agents. For example, heart failure is associated with Onglyza and Nesina. We do not know exactly if it is agent specific or if it is a class effect. Trajenta is not excreted through kidneys and does not have renal function limitations. I used it if the patient's insurance pays for it.

What should I know before I begin to take a DPP-4 inhibitor?

Here are seven things you need to know:

1. If you have a personal or family history of pancreatitis, pancreatic neoplasms or cancer, you should not take it.
2. If you have a very weak immune system-easily get all sorts of infection, discuss with your prescribing physician.
3. If you have a history of heart failure, especially active phase, it may not be a good idea to take it.
4. If you have poor renal function, the dose for Nesina, Januvia or Onglyza needs to be adjusted. Tradjenta doses do not need adjustment.
5. It is very rare, but it is reported that this group of medications, like other medication, might cause hypersensitivity, which can be life-threatening.
6. Although uncommon, cases of hepatic dysfunction have been reported in patients taking vildagliptin (I have never use it) and saxaglipitn.
7. DPP-4 inhibitors also have been associated with severe joint pain, especially Januvia and Onglyza. The real connection is not clear.

I heard that DPP-4 inhibitors cause heart failure. Is it true?

In April 2016, the FDA issued a label change for Onglyza and Nesina. These drugs might be associated with heart failure. It is still not clear if it is agent specific or a class effect.

When should I temporarily stop a DPP4-inhibitor?

If you have any of the following conditions, you should not take any DPP4-inhibitor:

1. You have pancreatitis or a family history of pancreatic cancer.
2. You are very sick with a fever and/or dehydration, especially if you have marginal kidney function or a history of heart failure.
3. You are not able to drink water or have severe nausea or vomiting.
4. You are on a metformin combination, and you are having a CT scan with contrast. Stop taking it 2-3 days before the CT scan. If your kidney function is marginal, I recommend you check your kidney function before you start taking it again.
5. You develop acute kidney failure.
6. You develop liver failure.
7. You are very sick and hospitalized.

What are GLP-1 agonists?

GLP-1 is a gut enzyme which has a series of effects on sugar homeostasis. It enhances glucose-dependent insulin secretion, slows gastric emptying, and reduces postprandial glucagon (glucagon is a hormone which can increase sugar) and helps to reduce food intake.

For now, they need to be injected.

What are the currently GLP-1 agonists on the market?

Currently, we have seven products in the US, and more may be in the pipeline.

1. Bydureon (exenatide) - taken once weekly
2. Byetta (exenatide) - taken twice daily
3. Trulicity (dulaglutide) - taken once weekly
4. Victoza (liraglutide) - taken once daily

5. IDegLira (Victoza+Tresiba) in Europe, Xultophy in the US. Tresiba is a long-acting insulin. This is very new. I have not used this product yet.
6. Tanzeum (albiglutide)- taken once weekly
7. SOLIQUA 100/33 combines Lantus, a long-acting insulin, with lixisenatide, a GLP-1 agonist, in a once daily shot. I started using it in February 2017. My patients seem to like it better having one shot a day instead of two shots.

Which GLP-1 agonist is the best?

It is very difficult to say. There are no head-to-head studies.

The efficacies are very similar. They can decrease HbA1c by 1-1.5%. Most patients have various degrees of weight loss (1.5 to 2.5 kg over 30 weeks). Some studies show that GLP-1 agonists might have favorable cardiovascular benefits.

If your insurance pays for everything, I like to use Trulicity which is the simplest device to give, and it is used only once a week.

Tanzeum is not too difficult either.

Victoza is a once-daily agent, and you can adjust the dose easily. The minimal FDA approved dose is 0.6, but I have been instructing patients to use 0.2 to 0.6 mcg daily if they have not been tolerating it due to gastrointestinal side effects.

Victoza is the first and only GLP-1 agent which showed favorable cardiovascular benefit.

How to adjust the dose of Victoza?

I also like Victoza. Although it is a once daily agent, it can be adjusted through a wide range of doses. It can be used in a wide range of renal functions. It can be stopped quickly in the case of side effects or if other conditions develop that require it to be stopped. The side effects are usually gone in a day.

I usually instruct patients to start with 0.6 mg before breakfast for one week, if tolerated, move it up to 1.2 mg the next week, and then to 1.8 mg daily. The point is to use the maximally tolerated dose. If a patient cannot tolerate 0.6 mg, I instruct the patient to try a smaller dose of 0.12 mg or 0.3 mg. There are no marks for these settings on the pen, but there is a way to do it. Between 0 to 0.6 mg there are 10 clicks. You can count 2 clicks (0.12 mg), you can count 5 clicks (0.3 mg). If you inject one click more or less, do not worry about it.

What should I know before I begin to take GLP-1 agonist?

These are the important things to keep in mind:

1. If you have a personal or family history of pancreatitis, pancreatic neoplasms or cancer, you should not take it.
2. If you have a very weak immune system and easily get all sorts of infections, discuss this with your prescribing physician.
3. If you have a history of heart failure, especially active phase, it may not be a good idea to take it.
4. If you have poor renal function, Byetta or Bydureon should not be used.
5. It is very rare, but it has been reported that this group of medications, like other medications, might cause hypersensitivity which can be life threatening
6. Family history of a rare thyroid cancer like medullary thyroid cancer or multiple endocrine neoplasia 2A or 2B.
7. GLP-1 agonists can be put on hold if you are severely sick, for example, if you have a fever, severe nausea, vomiting, and dehydration. Remember, it is okay to hold these drugs on occasions like these.
8. If you have a diagnosis of gastroparesis, you should not take it unless you specifically discuss this with your treating physician.

9. GLP-1 agonists are not insulin, but if you are using them with insulin or sulfonylurea or insulin releasing agents like glipizide, glimepiride or glyburide or glinides like Starlix, they can cause hypoglycemia. Therefore, the dose of insulin or sulfonylureas or glinides might need to be adjusted.

10. As we can see, now we have insulin and GLP-1 agonist combinations. If you are using Soliqua 100/33 or Xultophy, the combination of insulin and GLP-1 agonist, therefore the risk for low sugar is significantly increased.

11. GLP-1 agonists are proteins and might induce antibodies. Although in most cases this does not affect the efficacy or safety parameters, some patients develop high levels of antibodies that may decrease the glycemic response. If you think the effect of your medication is down, talk to your prescribing physician. He or she might be able to change the drug.

What should I do if I have too much nausea when I take a GLP-1 agonist?

Nausea is very common with the use of GLP-1 agonists.

According to prescribing information, nausea and vomiting rates for GLP-1 agonist are:

GLP-1 Agonist	Nausea	Vomiting
exenatide immediate-release (Byetta)	8%-44%	4-18%
exenatide extended-release (Bydureon)	11.3%-27%	10.8%-11.3%
liraglutide (Victoza)	7.5%-34.6%	6%-12.4%
Tanzeum	11%	4%

The most common adverse reactions reported in ≥5% of Trulicity-treated patients in placebo-controlled trials are:

Reaction	Placebo	Trulicity 0.75 mg	Trulicity 1.5 mg
nausea	5.30%	12.40%	21.10%
diarrhea	6.70%	8.90%	12.6%),
vomiting	2.30%	6.00%	12.70%

Nausea usually goes away in a week or two.

Always, start with the low dose and then advance to the higher dose. If you are using Victoza, you can reduce to 0.2 and then gradually advance the dose.

What is an SGLT2 inhibitor?

SGLT2 is a protein in humans that facilitates glucose reabsorption in the kidney. SGLT2 inhibitors block the reabsorption of glucose in the kidney, increase glucose excretion, and lower blood glucose levels. This is a new class of diabetes medication that can help you lose up to 100 g of sugar in the urine every day.

Which SGLT2 inhibitors are currently on the market?

Here are the seven medications on the US market, some with metformin or DPP-IV inhibitors:

1. Farxiga (dapagliflozin)
2. XigduoXR, Farxiga (dapagliflozin) with metformin extended release
3. Invokana (canagliflozin)
4. Invokamet, Invokana (canagliflozin) with metformin
5. Jardiance (empagliflozin)
6. Synjardy, Jardiance (empagliflozin) with metformin
7. Glyxambi, Jardiance (empagliflozin) Synjardy with Tradjenta.

Which SGLT2 inhibitor is the best?

Again, there are no head-to-head trials to prove which one is the best.

Doctors have to choose from your health insurance plan designations. Recently, Jardiance was shown to have cardiovascular benefits. It is not clear that the Jardiance effect is a drug class effect or just to Jardiance.

For the current three main agents, based on FDA approved prescription information, Jardiance also has an advantage with mild, renal impaired patients.

What should I know before I begin to take SGLT2 inhibitors?

You should know the following information before you take SGLT2 inhibitors:

1. The mechanism of this group of medication is to block the sugar reabsorption, so the sugar is removed in the urine. Just as in poorly controlled type 2 diabetes, the risk for UTIs and yeast infections is increased significantly.
2. Low blood pressure can occur. Loss of sugar also causes loss of water. If you do not drink enough water, you might feel dizziness and low blood pressure. If you are taking a diuretic, then you might need to adjust the dose or stop it. You might also need to adjust other blood pressure medications.
3. Again, if you are dehydrated, you might get an acute kidney injury.
4. In an Invokana clinical trial, the chances for bone fractures were increased. Bone fractures occur more frequently in patients taking canagliflozin (Invokana). I suspect this is caused by low blood pressure which caused the patients to fall. Therefore, it is very important that you drink plenty of water.
5. Patients treated with this group of medications are reported to be more prone to develop diabetic ketoacidosis. This is a serious

condition and can be life threatening. The exact mechanism is not known, but normal sugar levels delay the recognition of this condition by both the patient and physician.

6. In an ongoing trial with a mean of 4.5 years of follow-up, there were increases in leg and foot amputations (predominantly toes) in patients taking Invokana (7 versus 3 out of 1000 patients with 100 mg of Invokana and placebo respectively).

7. SGLT2 inhibitors can be put on hold if you are severely sick with symptoms of a fever, severe nausea, vomiting or dehydration. Remember, it is okay to put the medicine on hold during these occasions.

What can I do to reduce the chances for UTIs or yeast infections?

UTIs (urinary tract infections) and yeast infections are big issues for women. The chances of having these infections are very high. In clinical trials, they are reported at around 10%. In my experience, I think it is underreported.

Here is what you can do especially if you are a woman:

1. Drink lots of water, always bring water with you wherever you go. Every day, you need to drink at least 64 ounces of water.
2. Have two showers a day (morning and night).
3. Relieve yourself after sex.
4. Wash your private parts well after sex.

Does SGLT2 reduce cardiovascular risk in type 2 diabetes?

Some new data shows that SGLT2 might reduce cardiovascular risks in type 2 diabetes. The study repeated the results when empagliflozin (Jardiance) was added to standard care for type 2 diabetes patients at high cardiovascular risk. Jardiance produced a 38% relative risk reduction in cardiovascular mortality and a 32% risk reduction in all causes of mortality when compared with placebo among the patients with type 2 diabetes. All these patients had established cardiovascular disease and were already being treated with statins, angiotensin-converting inhibitors, and aspirin. SGLT2 revealed a 14% reduction for the combined risks of cardiovascular death, nonfatal MI, and nonfatal stroke.

Lawyers have Ads on TV, should I stop the medication?

No. Do not let a lawyer be your doctor. Let a doctor be your doctor. Listen to your doctor for medical advice and not a lawyer on TV.

When should I temporarily stop an SGLT2 antagonist?

If you have any of the following conditions, you should not take an SGLT2 antagonist;

1. You are very sick with fever and dehydration, especially if you have marginal kidney function or a history of heart failure.
2. You are not able to drink water or have severe nausea or vomiting.
3. You are on a metformin combination, and you are having a CT scan with contrast. Stop taking it 2-3 days before the CT scan. If your kidney function is marginal, I recommend you check your kidney function before you start taking it again.
4. You have acute kidney injury.
5. You have liver failure.
6. You have a urinary tract infection.
7. You are not able to drink water or if there is no place to go to the restroom.
8. You feel dizziness and your blood pressure is low. Certainly, you need to drink more water. You should then see your doctor for a medication adjustment.
9. You are diagnosed with bladder cancer or have a strong family history of bladder cancer.

10. You are frail or you do not want to lose weight.
11. You are very sick and hospitalized.

What is acarbose?

Most carbs you are eating cannot be absorbed directly. They need to be digested. Acarbose is called an alpha-glucosidase inhibitor. It blocks the gastrointestinal enzymes (alpha-glucosidase) that convert complex polysaccharide carbohydrates into monosaccharides that can be absorbed.

What are the adverse effects of acarbose?

GI (gastrointestinal) side effects are very common. It is reported that up to 73% of patients have excess flatulence and diarrhea.

How do I reduce the side effects of flatulence and diarrhea?

The only way to do it is to reduce your carb intake.

However, if you have some special social event to attend and excessive flatulence is not desirable, it is okay to miss the acarbose dose.

What should I do if I have lots of gas when I take acarbose?

See above. You can reduce the carb intake; you can reduce the medication intake. Sometimes, for important occasions when you are around many people, you can miss the dose.

When should I temporarily stop taking acarbose?

If you have any of the following conditions, you should not take acarbose:

1. You are very sick, with fever and dehydration, especially if you have marginal kidney function or a history of heart failure.
2. You are not able to drink water or have severe nausea or vomiting.
3. You have diarrhea.
4. You are bloated. Stop or reduce the dose.

5. You are on a metformin combination, and you are having a CT scan with contrast. Stop taking it 2-3 days before the CT scan. If your kidney function is marginal, I recommend you to check your kidney function before you start taking it again.
6. You are going to attend a social function and "gas" is not desirable.
7. You develop liver failure.
8. You are very sick and hospitalized.

I have type 2 diabetes, why does my doctor prescribe insulin for me?

Type 2 diabetes in the early stage is mainly caused by insulin resistance. However, at the time type 2 diabetes is diagnosed, it may already be in a later stage where there is more than 50% beta cell loss. Beta cells are the cells in the pancreas that secrete insulin. When the sugar is too high, it is toxic to the beta cells. It causes the remaining cells to die or malfunction. The use of insulin can preserve the remaining beta cells.

What is the best insulin that I should take for type 2 diabetes?

There is no best insulin to take.

For most cases, it is recommended that a basal insulin be started first since it is easy and it is only taken once or twice a day. Patients accept this very well.

We use so-called long-acting insulin as a basal insulin. These are Tresiba, Lantus, Toujeo, Levemir and biosimilar Basaglar. Sometimes, NPH can be used as a basal insulin.

What kind of insulin can I use for type 2 diabetes?

All kinds of insulin have been used in type 2 diabetes. As we discussed, basal insulins are usually used first. We start it once or twice a day depending on which basal insulin is chosen. Then, we start premeal insulin if we are not achieving our goal.

What should I know before I start insulin?

Here are several things you need to know before you start insulin:

1. Know the basics about insulin. Insulin is the hormone which is responsible to drive the glucose into cells to be metabolized. It will exert its function even when the sugar is already low.
2. Learning the concept of basal (long-acting) and bolus (fast-acting) insulin.
3. Long-acting-insulin usually works longer than 18 hours. It is taken once or twice a day. It starts to work in 1-2 hours.
4. Short-acting insulin starts to work in 15-30 minutes, and it lasts up to 4-5 hours. However, if you have poor renal function, your insulin might act longer, and you might need to reduce the dose.
5. Do not mistake the long-acting insulin for short-acting insulin and do not mistake short-acting insulin for long-acting insulin.
6. The risk for hypoglycemia is increased.
7. Learn the symptoms and signs for hypoglycemia and what to do if it happens.
8. Learn how to treat and prevent hypoglycemia.
9. Learn how to use the correction scale (sliding scale).
10. Learn the parameters to adjust the insulin dose.
11. Learn how to appropriately store the insulin.
12. Learn how to inject insulin.
13. Learn how to transport insulin.
14. Talk to your family about starting insulin and the risks for hypoglycemia.
15. Teach family members or friends who are living with you about your glucagon emergency kit and how to use it for hypoglycemia.
16. Check your sugar before you drive.

Should I give insulin before the meal or after the meal?

For basal (long-acting) insulin, you can give it at any time, before or after the meal. For once a day, it is better to take at the same time each day. For twice a day, take it 12 hours apart.

For bolus (short-acting insulin), it is recommended to take it before the meal. However, for some circumstances, we also recommend to take with or after the meal.

For example, if you do not have an appetite and do not know how much you are going to eat, it is recommended that you take your insulin immediately after the meal, or take it as soon as you know how much food you are going to consume.

Alternatively, for this circumstance described above, it is recommended that you take half of the dose before the meal, and then take half after you are able to finish your meal.

If your sugar is below 60-70, and if you do not have any low sugar symptoms, to be safe, we recommend you take your insulin after you start eating. Depending on how low the sugar is, you can reduce your dose by 20-80%.

Should I eat snacks on an insulin regimen?

When you take insulin, especially bolus insulin for your meals, snacks are not recommended. Since, when you snack, your next sugar check will be high since most people do not take insulin for snacks.

Some snacks are okay to eat such as no-carb snacks like cheese, or all vegetable snacks, or very low-carb snacks.

If you are snacking with some carbs, and you know how to do the carb count and know the carb ratio, you can give a bolus accordingly.

Your time between meals should not be more than 5 hours during the day. Five hours between meals is too long. You should plan your meals so that you eat four meals a day or three meals and a small snack. Your insulin regimen should be designed according to your meal times.

What should I do if I have low sugar?

Please see how to treat low sugar in the type 1 diabetes section.

What happened when my sugar is not low, but I feel like my sugar is low?

This is a complicated situation. This happens sometimes when your blood sugar has not been controlled for a long time, and then suddenly you take measures to lower your blood sugar. Your body is still used to high sugar, and now they are normal, but your body thinks it is too low. My recommendation is that at that moment you can eat something or treat it as low sugar to ease your symptoms.

I recommend you to correct your sugar slowly and then your body sense will be back to normal.

What is happening when I check my sugar and it is low, but I do not feel like it is low?

Here is two scenario. Your sugar shows below 60-70 but it may not be true. The meter is not so accurate at this level. Another scenario is hypoglycemia unawareness. Hypoglycemia unawareness is more common in long-term diabetes patients, but it can affect other patients as well. This can be a very distressing problem with diabetes. Normally, a person will feel warning symptoms when his or her blood sugar is low, such as shaking and sweating caused by the release of stress hormones like glucagon, cortisol, norepinephrine and epinephrine.

Serious problems can occur if this is not recognized and treated. Patients can lapse into a coma or have a grand mal seizure which can hurt them or other people depending what the patient is doing at that moment.

What can I do to recognize the hypoglycemia unawareness?

Please also review the section in type 1 diabetes.

Here are five things you can do.

1. Talk to your doctor about what is happening. He or she can adjust your medications.
2. Talk to your family, friends and coworkers to let them know if they notice you are acting weird or having some bizarre behavior, that they need to alert you to check your sugar.
3. If you pass out or a seizure occurs, have someone give you a glucagon shot right away even before calling 911.
4. The key to preventing this is to check your sugar more often.
5. If you are lucky enough to have an insurance to pay for CGM, this is highly recommended.

What bizarre behaviors do your friends and family need to pay attention to?

You need to tell your friends, family and coworkers that if you have these symptoms your sugar might be low. Tell them they need to alert you to check your sugar and treat it accordingly.

Here are the seven symptoms to watch for:

1. Irrational thoughts
2. Anger or irritability -- see also Anger During Lows
3. Running away
4. Insisting "I feel fine" in the midst of very unusual behavior
5. High stress
6. High emotions
7. Laughing and silliness

How do I regain hypoglycemia awareness?

Please also see the type 1 diabetes section.

The good news is that you can regain your hypoglycemia awareness by avoiding low sugar. Avoidance of low sugar enables people with diabetes to regain their symptoms when they become low. Here are four things you can do:

1. Set your goal or target to be higher than before. You need to call your doctor and tell him or her what is happening. He or she will carefully adjust your insulin doses or oral medications to closely match your diet and exercise regimen.
2. You should continue to be more alert to physical warnings for 48 hours following a low blood sugar episode.
3. Consider any blood sugar below 60 mg/dl (3.3 mmol) as serious and practice ways to avoid them.
4. Use your records to predict when lows are likely to occur.

Is CGM the best way to prevent hypoglycemia?

The technology is getting better and more accurate. I agree that CGM is the best technology you can have to prevent hypoglycemia. As long as you wear it, you can see the readings, and it will give you directions and warnings.

Chapter 9: All about insulin

Which type of insulin is best?

There is no best type. Every type of insulin has a different purpose for different people.

What is long-acting insulin?

Long-acting insulin starts in 1-2 hours and lasts at least 8 hours. We also call it basal insulin.

Here are the examples::

- NPH
- Levemir
- Lantus
- Basaglar (biosimilar Lantus)
- Toujeo
- Tresiba

What is fast-acting insulin?

Fast-acting is also known as rapid-acting insulin. It usually starts to act in 10-30 minutes and lasts 1-4 hours. We usually use it before meals or for the sliding scale (correction scale).

Currently these are on the market: Humulin R, Novolin R, Humalog, Novolog, Apidra. The latter three are analogs, and their onset of action is slightly faster than Humulin R or Novolin R. Strictly speaking, Humulin R and Novolin R are not fast-acting, but clinically, we use them as fast-acting. There is a faster insulin in development.

Are there any other types of insulin?

Other types of insulin include:

- Short-acting: all fast-acting insulins are short-acting. When some physicians discuss short-acting insulin, they are referring to Regular (R) Humulin R or Novolin R.
- Intermediate-acting insulin: NPH N.
- In this book, I use short-acting insulin, fast-acting insulin, bolus insulin interchangeably; I use long-acting insulin, slow-acting insulin, basal insulin interchangeably.
- Pre-mixed insulin. Premixed insulins combine specific amounts of intermediate-acting and short-acting/fast-acting insulin in one bottle or insulin pen. 75/25, 70/30 or 50/50 Humulin, Novolin, Humalog, or Novolog.
- Combination of long-acting (basal) insulin and GLP-1 agonist: Soliqua 100/33 is a combination of insulin glargine (Lantus) and the GLP-1 receptor agonist lixisenatide (Adlyxin in the US and Lyxumia in Europe). This can be used only for type 2 diabetes.
- Inhaled insulin. Afrezza is a rapid-acting (short-acting) inhaled insulin indicated to improve glycemic control in adult patients with diabetes mellitus. This was approved by FDA in 2014. It is a premeal insulin to be used on both type 1 and type 2 diabetes. In type 1 diaetes, Afrezza needs to be used with long-acting insulin.

Generic/Brand names for rapid-acting and short-acting insulins

Type of Insulin & Brand Names	Onset	Peak	Duration	Role in Blood Sugar Management
Rapid-Acting/Fast-Acting				
Lispro (Humalog)	15-30 min.	30-90 min	3-5 hours	Rapid-acting insulin covers insulin needs for meals eaten after the injection. This type of insulin is often used with long-acting insulin.
Aspart (Novolog)	10-20 min.	40-50 min.	3-5 hours	
Glulisine (Apidra)	20-30 min.	30-90 min.	1-2½ hours	
Short-Acting				
Regular (R) humulin or novolin	30 min. -1 hour	2-5 hours	5-8 hours	Short-acting insulin covers insulin needs for meals eaten within 30-60 minutes.

Brand names for intermediate-acting and long-acting insulins

Type of Insulin & Brand Names	Onset	Peak	Duration	Role in Blood Sugar Management
Intermediate-Acting				
NPH (N)- Novolin N, Humulin N	1-2 hours	4-12 hours	18-24 hours	Intermediate-acting insulin covers insulin needs for about half the day or overnight. This type of insulin is often combined with a rapid- or short-acting type.
Long-Acting				
Insulin glargine (Lantus)	1-1½ hours	No peak time. Insulin is delivered at a steady level.	20-24 hours	Long-acting insulin covers insulin needs for about one full day. This type is often combined, when needed, with rapid- or short-acting insulin in the regimen but not in the same injection.
Insulin glargine 3X (toujeo)	1-2 hours	No peak; at steady level	24-36 hours	
Insulin degludec (Tresiba)	1-2 hours	No peak; at steady level	36-48 hours	
Insulin detemir (Levemir)	1-2 hours	6-8 hours	Up to 24 hours	

Brand names for premixed insulins

Type of Insulin & Brand Names	Onset	Peak	Duration	Role in Blood Sugar Management
Pre-Mixed*				
Humulin 70/30	30 min.	2-4 hours	14-24 hours	These products are generally taken two or three times a day before mealtime.
Novolin 70/30	30 min.	2-12 hours	Up to 24 hours	
Novolog 70/30	10-20 min.	1-4 hours	Up to 24 hours	
Humulin 50/50,	30 min.	2-5 hours	18-24 hours	
Humalog mix 75/25, Humalog 50/50	15 min.	30 min.-2½ hours	16-20 hours	

*Premixed insulins combine specific amounts of intermediate-acting and short-acting/rapid-acting insulin in one bottle or insulin pen. The numbers following the brand name indicate the percentage of each type of insulin.

Who can use inhaled insulin?

As indicated by FDA, Afrezza can be used both in adult type 1 and type 2 diabetes patients. It is contraindicated if you are a smoker or you have COPD or asthma or other chronic lung disease. I also recommend you use other forms of insulin if you have respiratory infection.

What should I do if I forget long-acting insulin?

This depends on what you are taking and how often you are taking it.

1. If you are taking Tresiba, you usually are asked to take it once a day in the morning or night. If you forget one dose, you can take it as soon as possible. You can go back to the regular schedule of injections as long as your next regularly scheduled injection is at least 12 hours away. If your regularly scheduled injection is within 12 hours, you can give one shot as soon as possible, then give another shot after 12 hours, then go back to your regular schedule.
2. If you are taking Lantus (biosimilar Basaglar) or Toujeo, you are probably taking it once a day. If you forget one dose, catching up is more complicated. If the next dose is still 12 hours away, I recommend that you take half a dose to catch up. If your next dose is less than 12 hours away but more than 8 hours away, you can choose to take a third of your usual dose to catch up or just miss a dose. If the next dose is less than 8 hours away, just miss a dose but give the next shot 2 hours earlier than your usual time. Whatever you do, you need to check your sugar and give correction if needed.
3. If you are taking Levemir once a day, follow 2 above.
4. If you are taking Levemir or Lantus (or Basaglar) twice a day, you can take a dose as soon as you can. Then, you can push your next dose back by 2 hours, and then your next dose by 1 hour, and then back to your usual schedule. For example, if you give yourself insulin everyday at 9 am and 9 pm and you forget your morning dose until noon, you can give it at noon. Based on the schedule of every 12 hours, your next dose should be midnight, but you need to move 2 hours ahead, which would make it 10pm. The next day, you can return to your regular schedule of 9 am and 9 pm. If you only forget within 2 hours of your normally scheduled time, you can keep your normal schedule without corrections. If you miss your Levemir or Lantus, and you do not have it, then you may just

have to wait until your next dose. If you have fast-acting insulin, you can give fast-acting insulin based on the sliding scale.

5. If you are taking NPH every 12 hours, you can follow the same correction as Levemir.
6. If you are taking pre-mixed insulin, and It is much more complicated, you should be better call your doctor for advice.

What should I do if I accidentally inject fast-acting insulin for long-acting insulin?

Sometimes distinguishing long-acting and short-acting insulin can be confusing. I often get calls about what to do if you mixed up the long-acting and fast-acting insulin.

Here is what you need to do:

1. Do not panic.
2. Depending on your sugar level and insulin sensitivity, your reaction to this mistake is unique.
3. Eat a regular meal and give half of the dose of long-acting insulin. If you have the correct dose and regimen, your sugar should continue to be stable. If you are prone to have low sugar, check your sugar every 2 hours to make sure it is stable.
4. If you are in a situation, in which you do not have a meal to eat, you can miss one dose of long-acting insulin. Check your sugar every 1-2 hours to make sure you are not developing low sugar. If you develop low sugar, treat accordingly.
5. If you are alone and you do not have anything to eat, and you cannot check your sugar, call 911 as soon as possible.

What should I do if I accidentally inject long-acting insulin for fast-acting insulin?

It is slightly more challenging in this case, but there is no need to panic. The chances of you developing low sugar is much lower compared to the mistake of injecting fast-acting for long-acting because the fast-acting dose is usually only one third of a long-acting dose.

1. If this happens during the day, you may just omit the fast-acting for the meal. Your sugar will go up, but that is fine. Then, reduce your fast-acting insulin by half for the day. Again, your sugar might be high for a day, but it is fine. It is important in this situation to make sure your sugar is not low.
2. If you are prone to have low sugar and your next meal is 5-6 hours away, you might need to check your sugar in 4 hours to make sure your sugar is not low.
3. Check your sugar at midnight to make sure it is not low.
4. If you make the mistake at night, again, just to be safe, omit your fast-acting insulin. Your sugar should go up at bedtime instead of going down, but it is fine to have high sugar for one day.
5. Check your sugar at midnight to make sure it is not going too low. If it is, eat a snack, then reduce your second daytime fast-acting insulin by half. Again, your sugar may go up, but this is safer than going down.
6. If you are trying to get your sugar perfect even in this situation, you can give half or two-thirds of your pre-meal insulin again, and continue your long-acting schedule if the next long-acting is normally your next dose. If your next long-acting dose is less than 12 hours away, please reduce it by one-third (the amount you have given already).

What should I do if I accidentally inject myself with long-acting as short-acting and short-acting as long-acting?

Things can happen. There is no need to panic.

Some patients have both long-acting and short-acting insulin shots at the same time in the morning, which is no problem. Normally, the long-acting dose is three times more than the short-acting dose, so you have given yourself three times as much of the short-acting dose and one-third of the normal long-acting dose.

In the morning, your sugar may go down because you have too much short-acting insulin. Therefore, you need to eat more for your breakfast. However, for lunch and dinner, if you give yourself the correct dose, then your pre-meal or midnight sugar may go up. You might need to give more sliding scale.

Check your sugar one more time between the meal and midnight to make sure your sugar is not too low or too high. If you follow this schedule, your sugar may be slightly elevated, which is good in this case. After 24 hours, then go back to your regular schedule.

If you are in this situation, and if you still want to be perfect, you can eat twice as much for the meal and give 2/3 of the long-acting basal insulin again. Continue the insulin regimen as usual. Again, it is very important to check your sugar.

Why is pre-mixed insulin not optimal for type 1 diabetes?

Now we have analog pre-mixed insulin and regular fast-insulin pre-mixed.

For Humalog, we have a Humalog mix with NPH 50:50 (Humalog 50% and NPH 50%); we also have Humalog mix with NPH 75:25 (NPH 75% and Humalog 25%).

For Novolog mix with NPH70:30 (Novolog 30% and NPH 70%).

For regular fast-insulin, we have NPH mixed with Humulin R or Novolin R 70/30 (70% NPH and 30% of regular insulin).

The benefit of pre-mixed is that it is one shot for both fast- and long-acting insulin. There are analog premix insulin and regular premix insulin. The regular premix insulin is more affordable.

Disadvantages for pre-mixed insulin:

1. The ratio for fast-acting and long-acting is fixed. You cannot change it as needed.
2. The effect for both fast and long-acting insulin has been changed, which increases the risk for too low or too high sugar.
3. Pre-mixed insulin is not easy to adjust.
4. Pre-mixed insulin varies widely and needs to be mixed very well before usage.

Why are some insulins clear and other insulins cloudy?

Any insulin with NPH is cloudy. These are Novolin N, Humulin N, and any pre-mixed insulin.

How should I store insulin?

1. For unused insulin vials or pens, they should be stored in a refrigerator and never frozen. They can be stored until the expiration date on the vials or pens.
2. For a used vial, you can store at room temperature or store it in the refrigerator. Either way, it does not affect its potency. However, if you store it in the refrigerator, it is recommended to allow it to warm up to room temperature before giving the injection. This reduces irritation at the injection site.
3. If you start to use the vial, the storage life ranges from seven days to one month depending on the brand. Please check the product package.
4. For pens, after you start using them, do not put them back into the refrigerator. Keep them at room temperature. The following list details common brand storage life:
    - Humalog 100 or 200 (28 days)
    - Humulin N (14 days)Humalog mix 75/25 (10 days)
    - Humalog mix 50/50 (10 days)
    - Humulin mix 75/25 (10 days)

- Novolin R (28 days)
- Novolin N (14 days)
- Novolin 70/30 (10 days)
- Novolog (28 days)
- Toujeo (28 days)
- Tresiba (8 wks)
- Lantus/Basaglar (28 days)

I do not have a good memory. I think I gave myself a shot a minute ago, but I am not sure if I did or did not. Is there anything I can do?

Insulin can be very dangerous. If this is the case for you, I would recommend that you discuss with your prescribing doctor if it is possible to not to use insulin in your regimen.

If you must use insulin, timer caps are available for your insulin pen. Every time you put on the cap, it starts a timer, so that you can see the last time you used the pen. This prevents you from injecting yourself twice. The timer cap is called a Timsulin smart pen cap. You can Google it or buy it from Kmart.

Which one is better? Pen or vial?

I like pens better, because you do not have to draw the insulin. It is much easier, especially for the elderly. Pens are also more convenient to use when you go out to eat. They can easily fit in your purse or pocket.

Which needle is better?

Most needles do not cause any pain. Use the smallest needle possible. My patients have reported that Novofine Plus is very good.

Shunzhong Shawn Bao, M.D.

Where can I inject?

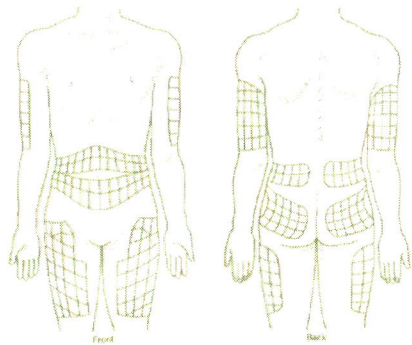

Common insulin injection sites

What else do I need to remember when I do an injection?

1. Only use injection sites that are smooth, with no signs of infection, bumps, or scars.
2. Always rotate the injection site.
3. If you take long-acting insulin, you can inject it on your thigh at night, because you will not be active. Movement and exercise can affect insulin absorption, so you need to be as consistent as possible.
4. Some patients use rotation tattoos, because it helps them keep track of injection sites.

If I have type 2 diabetes. What can I do to prevent weight gain with insulin use?

Insulin is an anabolic hormone, meaning it helps synthesize the building blocks of your body, causing you to gain weight. Most patients on insulin gain weight. But if you take the following measures, you do not need to gain weight.

1. Try not to eat snacks while you are on insulin. Many doctors will ask you to eat snacks to prevent low sugar, but this is wrong.

Eating more snacks will cause you to have a higher chance of having low sugar, because when you check your sugar, it will always be high. If your sugar is always high, your doctor will increase your insulin dose, because your sugar is not controlled, and you will gain more weight.

2. Try to use the lowest dose possible (for type 2 diabetes). Type 1 diabetes is more complicated. You need to talk to your doctor specifically about this issue.
3. Focus on lifestyle changes.
4. I recommend that you do some sort of exercise before each meal, which will increase your insulin sensitivity, and your need for insulin will decrease.
5. Cut down fat intake. Fat decreases your insulin sensitivity and then your dose will need to be increased.
6. Cut down on carbs.
7. Ask your doctor if you qualify to use insulin in combination with some newer diabetes medications which can help you lose weight. There are the medications: GLP-1 agonists like Byetta, Byduren, Trulicity, Tanzeum, and Victoza; or SGLT2 antagonists like Farxiga, Invokana, and Jardiance, as well as their combinations.
8. Ask your doctor to review your medication list to see if you can get off medications that cause weight gain.

Do you have general tips on how to use insulin?

These general insulin shot recommendations are for fixed dose patients.

Maintain a routine of three meals every day and be as consistent as possible with the amount of carbohydrates in each meal. A small snack might be necessary in between meals and at bedtime (see a dietician). Exercise helps you burn calories, especially carbohydrates and sugar. A 20-30 minute walk after or before a meal is a good idea! **Keep a written record** of meals, sugar numbers, etc.! You might need to reduce your premeal insulin if you plan to exercise before or after the meal (see the exercise section).

Other important tips:

1. Make sure to give yourself short-acting insulin 15-20 minutes before you eat.
2. Check your sugar before you give short-acting insulin. You can adjust your dose based on your sugar numbers. Keep your correcting/sliding scale handy, so you can adjust your insulin doses.
3. Long-acting, Lantus, Basaglar, Toujeo, Levemir, Tresiba is to be injected at the same time every day (usually morning or at bedtime). Tresiba can be injected as a "catch up"—I recommend that you stick to the schedule.
4. ROTATE injection sites as instructed!
5. Physical activity lowers your blood sugar. Check your blood sugar before engaging in strenuous physical activities. Anaerobic exercise will decrease your sugar faster. You need to be more vigilant when you are engaging in anaerobic exercise.
6. You must establish a meal routine (three meals daily) and remain consistent in the amount of carbohydrates as well as controlling your portion sizes. If you would like to eat three meals plus one snack, that is fine. Talk to your doctor, so your regimen can be changed accordingly.
7. Insulin is a treatment, not a cure! DO NOT RELY ON INSULIN ALONE! Healthy eating, physical activity, keeping a record, and testing are the keys.
8. DO NOT STOP injecting insulin without consulting your doctor and/or diabetes educator.
9. Check your sugar before you drive, and always keep some sugar or snacks in your car or purse in case of emergency.

Can you tell me more about basal and bolus regimen?

Usually, you are prescribed two kinds of insulin, long-acting and short-acting. The long-acting insulins (Lantus, Basaglar, Toujeo, Levemir, Tresiba) serve as basal insulin to be taken once or twice a day. Therefore, in discussion, we consider long-acting insulin, basal insulin, and slowacting insulin interchangeable; we consider short-acting insulin and fast-acting insulin interchangeable.

The basal insulin is used to control fasting sugar between meals. We usually adjust your basal insulin based on fasting sugar.

The fast-acting insulin (Humalog, Novolog, Apida, Humulin R and Novolin R) is taken before each meal. This is your bolus insulin. They are for meals. You need to adjust your fast-acting insulin based on your post meal sugar. You can adjust both long-acting and short-acting. Usually, we recommend adjusting fast-acting insulin (bolus) more than the long-acting insulin (basal).

What is a sliding scale? How do I use it?

The sliding scale is called a correction scale. When you take fast-acting insulin, we usually use the correction scale to correct high sugar. The idea is to get your sugar down by injecting fast-acting insulin based on the scale.

Different patients need different scales. You need to discuss with your doctor what correction scale you need to use. I usually print a scale for my patients.

I have type 1 diabetes. Do you have general recommendations about how to adjust long-acting insulin?

Life is complicated, and type 1 diabetes and insulin can make your life even more complicated. These are my general recommendations, although you need to speak to your doctor.

1. If you are giving long-acting insulin in the morning, and if your sugar is >80 in the morning, and if you are very healthy and do not get low sugar easily, you can give a full dose of long-acting insulin. If your sugar is below 60, then you might need to eat something first and then give half of the dose. If your sugar is between 60 and 80, you can give half of your long-acting insulin dose. It is important that you need to seek more specific advice from your doctor for your particular situation.
2. If you are giving your long-acting insulin at night, and if your sugar is >130 at bedtime, you can give the full dose. If your sugar is between 100 and 130, you might need to cut down your night time long-acting insulin by half or 1/3. If your sugar is below 100, then you might need to eat a small snack and then give a half dose of long-acting insulin.
3. If you have frequently high or low sugar, you need to talk to your doctor. Your insulin regimen might need to be adjusted.

I have type 2 diabetes. Do you have a general recommendation about how to adjust long-acting insulin?

If you are relatively healthy, and if you do not get hypoglycemic easily, you can follow the recommendations I gave for type 1 diabetes above.

If you have multiple comorbidities or are very fragile, I would raise your sugar slightly. If your bedtime sugar is above 160, you can give the full dose. If it is between 130 and 160, you can consider half of the dose. If it is below 130, then you can omit the dose completely.

Is there an app to help me to calculate my insulin dosage?

When we use apps or machines, we tend to trust the machine more than our own instincts. If you take an overdose of insulin, it could kill you. Therefore, unless your doctor is familiar with the particular app, I do not recommend that you use it. I have a patient who uses an old insulin pump to calculate his insulin dosage. I put in all the settings, and he uses it to calculate his bolus.

What should I do with those needles and sharps?

You know you should not throw away your sharps into regular trash, but you might not know what to do with them. In America, every community has a Community Sharps Collection Program. The Community Sharps Collection Program usually provides a free container. If you do not know of a program, you can ask your doctor.

You can go to this website (http://www.safeneedledisposal.org/) to locate the nearest location for a sharp disposal site. You can also call 1-800-643-1643 to find a location.

If your community does not have one, you can ask your doctor for a container or buy one from target or Wal-Mart and bring it back to your doctor's office when it is full.

There are also sharp disposal mail programs. You can try Pureway Sharps Disposal System (pureway.com), GRP Sharps Disposal (sharpsdisposal.com), or Sharps Compliance (sharpsinc.com).

You might also contact your local health department for further information.

Chapter 10: Let's talk more about eating

What can I eat?

This is too big a question to answer. However, you can eat anything you want to eat; but certainly, you cannot eat the same way you have in the past. You need to change how much you eat, how you prepare your food, what you eat, when you eat, and what foods to eat together. A dietician can help you learn all this.

Again, there is nothing you cannot eat. It is recommended that you stay away from foods with high sugar and carbs. You need to avoid refined carbs and large amounts of food. I have a table to help you choose what to eat in the first part of Chapter 1.

Can I eat fruit? Which ones are the best?

The answer is certainly yes, but you cannot eat too much. We always say, "fruit is good for you." Fruit is loaded with vitamins, minerals, and fiber just like vegetables. But, fruit is not the same as vegetables. Fruit has too much sugar.

Tropical fruit is not recommended. This includes bananas(1/2 is okay), and pineapples., Some bananas are okay, if they are not too sweet. Papayas are okay.

Eat more vegetables instead of fruits. You should eat cucumbers, tomatoes, carrots, mushrooms, cauliflower, broccoli and celery.

Please read the previous questions about diet and how you should be eating.

Here is the fruit I recommended to my patients the most. Remember, portion control is still very important.

Berries

Blackberries and blueberries are the best. They have low sugar content and might have antioxidants. Raspberries are also very good. The have very low carbohydrates. Cranberries are good, too. Strawberries are not the best, but 3-5 are okay. They can be too sweet.

Goji Berries

I have never seen fresh Goji berries in stores. You can buy them from a Chinese store. They are very low in carbs. In Chinese medicine, they are used to increase sexual vitality. They have lots of antioxidants.

Apples

Most apples are okay for you to have one a day. Eat an apple a day, keep the doctor away! However, Fuji apples are too sweet for you.

Peaches

Some peaches can be too sweet for you. One a day is okay.

Tart cherries

Tart cherries are low in sugar. One cup is fine for you.

Cantaloupe

Some cantaloupe are okay too. One cup is maximum.

Papayas

Papayas are good.

Kiwis, Plums, Apricots and Avocados

These are all good.

What are the best vegetables for diabetes?

All non-starchy vegetables are good for diabetes. Here is a list of the most common.

Recommended fresh vegetable list

amaranth greens (Chinese spinach)	greens (collard, kale, mustard, turnip)
artichoke	hearts of palm
artichoke hearts	jicama (Mexican turnips)
asparagus	kohlrabi (German cabbage)
baby corn	leeks
bamboo shoots	mushrooms
beans (green, wax, Italian)	okra
bean sprouts	onions
beets	pea pods
Brussels sprouts	peppers
broccoli	radishes
cabbage	rutabaga
bok choy (Chinese cabbage)	salad greens (chicory, endive, escarole, lettuce, romaine, spinach, arugula, radicchio, watercress)
carrots	sprouts
cauliflower	squash (cushaw, summer, crookneck, spaghetti, zucchini)
celery	sugar snap peas
chayote squash	Swiss chard
coleslaw (packaged, no dressing)	tomatoes
cucumbers	turnips
daikon (Chinese radish)	water chestnuts
eggplant	yard-long beans

I have heard that green tea is good for me. Can drinking green tea help reduce my hunger? When should I drink it?

Green tea is very popular in China. Many health benefits have been claimed with drinking green tea.

Green tea is believed to aid in weight loss, lower cholesterol, and have an antioxidant effect. However, it is really hard to do clinical trials to prove all these good effects.

I, myself, drink green tea. It is safe to drink. You can try it yourself to see what kind of effect it has on you.

Drinking tea also provides you with adequate hydration that is good for your diabetes and weight loss.

You can drink green tea at any time of the day. However, since tea is a stimulant which might affect your sleep, I would not recommend that you drink it at night.

What are your favorite foods, and how do you prepare them?

Asparagus

Asparagus is my number one favorite. When I am home alone, this is the one dish I go to. It is so easy to prepare. I sometimes grill, bake, or just pan-fry it. In reality, I do pan-fry more often. I just cut off the dry ends, and then rinse them. I add some vegetable oil in the pan to grease the pan, add a little water, put in the asparagus, put it on the stove and turn on the heat. That is it. After you see the steam coming out of the pan, you just stir a few times until it is dry (do not add too much water—otherwise it will never dry). That is it.

Celery

My second favorite is celery. Most of the time, I just boil it until it soft, and then I add some soy sauce. Sometimes, I cook it with tofu. I boil celery as above and cook my tofu separately. Then I mix them together with some olive oil. You can add some black pepper or any other spices if you like.

Carrots and daikon soup

My third favorite is carrots and daikon soup. American soup is mostly cream based or broth based. It either has too much salt or too much fat. This soup is good. It does not have fat, and it does not have too much salt. You just cut some daikon and carrots into cubes, add a few dried shrimp (you can buy them from an Asian grocery store), add an appropriate amount of water and boil until soft. You can eat this before your meal to curb your appetite. You can also use it as a snack.

Spinach

Another of my favorites is spinach. I eat it by itself or with bean sprouts. You can eat it raw, but I prefer to stir-fry it with a few drops of vegetable oil.

Zucchini

There is nothing easier than cooking zucchini. You can cut zucchini into whatever shape you like. Just stir and fry. It is also easy to grill.

Chicken broccoli

You might have been to a Chinese restaurant and had chicken broccoli. I usually use chicken breasts which are easy to deal with. I cook the broccoli and chicken breast separately. I just cut the chicken into small pieces. Then, I add some chicken seasoning from Sam's Club with garlic. It just takes a few minutes to cook the chicken breasts. I cut the broccoli into pieces, and just boil them until they are a little soft (not too long, otherwise, it will be too soft). Then, I just mix them. You can add salt if you want.

Onions and mushrooms

I use whatever onions I have and cut them into pieces. I stir and fry the onions until soft. I add the pieces of mushrooms and stir and fry for one or two more minutes.

Okra

I love okra. It is so easy to cook. You can stir fry it with minimal oil, you can just boil it, or you can grill it. You can also bake it to make vegetable chips.

Green beans

They are so easy to prepare, just like okra. You can boil them. I like to stir fry or grill them.

Tomato egg soup

Nothing is easier to cook than this soup. You just cut a tomato, put it into boiled water until it boils again. Then add a beaten egg and stir a few times with a spoon. Add whatever seasoning you like. This soup is good to curb your appetite.

Baked or steamed squash such as acorn squash

Squash like acorn squash have lots of vitamins and fiber. It is very easy to cook. I just cut them into pieces and rinse off the seeds and bake them or steam them. You can season with anything you like. The carbs are low. I use them to replace my carbs from potato, rice or bread.

What are your recommendations for breakfast?

Everybody says that breakfast is very important. I get lots of questions about what to eat for breakfast. Most breakfast foods have too much sugar, too many carbs, and too much fat.

Here are the foods I recommend for breakfast. You can make different combinations if you like:

1. Good fruit and berries, as we discussed in the fruit section. I like blackberries, blueberries, cranberries, strawberries, kiwi, guava, cherries, pears, peaches, cantaloupe — with most of them you still need to practice portion control. Fruit has a lot fructose and they are sugar. You can eat them whole, or you can make smoothies.

2. Greek yogurt. Some versions of Greek yogurt have too much sugar. You need to look at them. On top of the yogurt you can add some chia seeds to add some texture to it. Chia seeds also add extra protein and fiber. You can also try adding some flaxseeds onto your yogurt. Flaxseeds have lots of omega-3 oil and magnesium.

3. Try some beans and lentils to replace animal proteins. There are lots of different ways to prepare beans. They are high in protein and relatively low in carbs. They are good replacements for pure carbs. You can buy or make chickpea hummus to eat with whole wheat bread. Edamame can be consumed at any time of the day.

4. Use whole grains to replace refined carbs. You can try barley or buckwheat. You can just boil them or slow cook them overnight. They have lots of magnesium which might help some people relieve leg cramps. Whole grain rye bread is also a better choice.

5. Oatmeal is often recommended. Overnight oats are a good choice. You can put oats, nuts and some milk in a jar and leave it in the refrigerator overnight. You can eat it in the morning.

6. Oat bran flakes are an alternative if you need a quick and easy breakfast.

7. Some whole grain cereal is acceptable.
8. Quinoa is also a good choice. It has good protein and fiber. The only thing you need to do is to boil it. Quinoa pasta is also good for dinner.
9. Small amounts of cheese. If you are not picky, you can try some vegetables with cottage cheese in the morning.
10. Eggs. I usually recommend no more than one egg a day, but you might eat a few egg whites in a day.

What are some of your ideas about snacks?

Now, you know already that I do not recommend snacks, especially if you are on insulin. I am talking about snacking when your sugar is not low. I divide snacks into three tiers: first tier, second tier and third tier. I prefer first-tier.

What are your first-tier snacks?

I recommend first-tier snacks like vegetables. These are low-carb, low-calorie snacks like broccoli, celery, cauliflower, and tomatoes. I also put carrots in this category. In this tier of snacks, you do not really need to worry about portion control. However, do not use dips.

What are your second-tier snacks?

I put low-carb, low-calorie snacks into this tier like nuts (almonds, walnuts, peanuts, pistachios, hazelnuts, cashews, Brazil nuts, pecans). Seaweed is a low-carb, low-calorie snack, but I put it in this tier due to the fact that if you buy it from an Asian store, it has too much salt and oil. If you prepare it yourself, I would put it in the first tier. Some protein bars can be in this tier. I put protein bars in this tier since they have their own portion control. I do not expect you to eat more than one.

What are your third-tier snacks?

I put moderate-carb snacks with a few calories into this tier. You really need to have portion control. Examples are edamame, pumpkin seeds, and cheese. Some good fruit like blackberries, blueberries, and raspberries are third-tier.

What is the best dressing I can use?

We know that salads are good for you, but there are two pitfalls of which you need to be aware.

1. Do not load your salad with high-fat ingredients like lots of cheese, bacon, and croutons.
2. Do not soak your salad in unhealthy dressings. If you do not pay attention to the amount of fat in the dressing, you can defeat the purpose of eating salads.

So, what are the best salad dressings to use? The fact is that you can use any of your favorite dressings. The key is how much and how you use it.

I recommend you put your salad dressing on the side and only use your fork to dip into it. You can dip it once with each mouthful of salad. Be assured, you can use any dressing you like. You are eating healthy. As every food, portion control is always the key.

If you are one of those people who always like plenty of choices, you can choose any dressing. Just limit yourself to two tablespoons. Just be sure the calories are less than 50 and the salt is less than 300 mg.

Salad dressing list

Here is a list of salad dressings I have compiled for you:

	Calories	Fat g	Sat fat g	Cholesterol	Sodium mg	Carbs g	Sugar g	Protein g	Comments
Bernstein's									
Light Fantastic Parmesan Garlic Ranch	50	2.5	0.5	5	330	6	2	1	slightly high in sodium
Dorothy Lynch									
Fat-Free Dressing	55				180	12	10	2	Slightly high in calories and sugar.
Hidden Valley									
Greek Yogurt Cucumber Dill	60	5	1		240	3	2	1	Slightly high in calories
Fiesta Salsa Ranch Light	60	5	1		240	3	1		Slightly high in calories
Pomegranate Vinaigrette	60	6			100	3	2		Slightly high in calories

	Calories	Fat g	Sat fat g	Cholesterol	Sodium mg	Carbs g	Sugar g	Protein g	Comments
Ken's Steak House									
Light Olive Oil & Vinegar	50	4	0.5		240	3	3		
Kraft									
Lite Balsamic Vinaigrette	25	1			210	4	4		
Lite Asian Toasted Sesame	45	1.5		10	260	7	6		
Lite Raspberry Vinaigrette	30	1			240	5	5		
Litehouse									
Lite Ranch	60	5		10	210	3	2	1	Slightly high in calories
Siracha Lime	20				200	5	5		
Mango Habanero	25				170	6	5		
Sesame ginger	40				270	9	8		

	Calories	Fat g	Sat fat g	Cholesterol	Sodium mg	Carbs g	Sugar g	Protein g	Comments
Pear Gorgonzola Vinaigrette	50	2.5			240	7	6		
Maple Grove Farms of Vermont									
Fat Free Balsamic Vinaigrette	15				120	3	2		
Fat Free Cranberry Balsamic Vinaigrette	35				220	8	7		
Fat Free Honey Dijon	40				210	10	9	1	
Lite Caesar	50	4.5			260	4	3		
Marie's									
Balsamic Vinaigrette	45	4.5			220	2	2		
Raspberry Vinaigrette	50	3			100	7	6		

	Calories	Fat g	Sat fat g	Cholesterol	Sodium mg	Carbs g	Sugar g	Protein g	Comments
Trader Joe's									
Raspberry Vinaigrette	40	3			60	4	4		
Fat Free Balsamic Vinaigrette	25				170	6	5		
Sesame Soy Ginger Vinaigrette	35				230	9	8		

Walden Farms-seems to have 0 calories and around 260 mg salt

Wish Bone Fat-Free - below 50 calories and around 300 mg of salt.

When is the best time to eat fruit?

You can eat fruit before or after you exercise.

You can eat fruit immediately after a meal as the dessert if you are on insulin. Your insulin will work on the carbs from the fruit.

If your sugar is not under good control, I do not recommend fruit for you.

What can I eat if my doctor does not recommend fruit for me?

Eat more vegetables instead of fruit. You should eat cucumbers, tomatoes, carrots, mushrooms, cauliflower, broccoli and celery.

Can I eat sugar-free cookies?

We talked about sugar substitute separately. Sugar-free is not carb free. Cookies may say no added sugar, but they still have many carbs you need to consider.

Can I eat sugar-free ice cream?

Again, sugar-free is not carb free. If you eat one cup, you still have around 30 g of carbs, and 8 g of fat.

How many carbohydrates may I eat?

I recommend a low-carb diet. A very low-carb diet is typically taking 50 grams per day. However, I do not recommend carbs just on face value. Not all carbs are the same, and the food you eat with the carbs also makes a difference to your blood sugar. It is not just how many carbs you eat, it is the kind of carbs you eat, and the other kinds of food you eat with them.

I recommend no refined and processed carbs like white rice and white bread. If these are the only carbs you have, I recommend you eat lots of vegetables first and then eat these carbs. Vegetables are low in carbs and high in fiber. There are no limits on the amount of vegetables you can eat. Beans are high in carbs, but their effect on blood sugar is much less profound. You still need to practice portion control on beans.

Should I calculate my calories every day?

There are ways to calculate the calories. I see a lot of apps that can calculate daily calories for you. However, in the long term, these calculations do not work. The reason is that life is more complicated than calculations. We just eat what we have, and we cannot calculate first and then eat. Moreover, those calculations are not accurate anyway. Our body can adjust our expenditures along with the calorie intake.

What is the best diet?

There really is no "best diet." It is a lifestyle change. However, I have a "best diet" that I recommend. On this diet you do not have to count calories. In my life, I have never seen a real vegetarian who is overweight. I cannot say that they do not have diabetes. At the same time, I believe in a balanced diet. Therefore, I recommend that my patients strive to be a borderline vegetarian.

People say fiber is good for diabetes. How much fiber should I consume every day?

Fiber is good. Studies show that enough fiber actually reduces the postprandial sugar. It also lowers the risk of cancer, lowers blood pressure, lowers blood cholesterol and lowers the risk of cardiovascular disease.

Again, I do not recommend that you count your fiber. If you follow the plant-based diet I recommend, you will get more than you need.

What is a low-fat diet? Is it good for diabetes?

A low-fat diet is a diet that reduces the daily intake of fat to 30% of caloric intake or less. Some studies show that a low-fat diet helps people lose more weight in comparison to a standard diet (usually 35-40% of fat). Since the fat in most low-fat diets is substituted with more carbs, this is not good for controlling diabetes.

What is the DASH diet? Is it good for diabetes?

DASH stands for Dietary Approaches to Stop Hypertension. As you can see this diet was initially designed for hypertension. This diet plan is rich in fruit, vegetables, whole grains, lean protein and low-fat dairy, and light on sugar, sodium, and fatty red meats. The DASH diet encourages you to reduce the sodium in your diet and eat a variety of foods rich in nutrients that help lower blood pressure, such as potassium, calcium and magnesium. It can also help your weight. If you reduce the portions and stick to it, you can also lower your HbA1c. Therefore, it is not a bad diet to follow.

What is the Mediterranean diet? Is it good for diabetes?

The Mediterranean Diet is a way of eating based on the traditional food (and drinks) of the countries surrounding the Mediterranean Sea. Most healthy diets include fruit, vegetables, fish and whole grains, and limit unhealthy fats. The Mediterranean diet also focuses on plant-based vegetables and fruit. The diet replaces butter with healthy fats such as olive oil and canola oil. It uses herbs and spices instead of salt to flavor food. It limits eating red meat to no more than a few times a month. It recommends eating fish and poultry at least twice a week. It is not a bad diet to follow for diabetes.

Are there any other diets I can follow?

There are many other diets. I think we have too many diets. I still believe that portion control is the key. Start thinking of yourself more as a vegetarian. Then, you do not need to think too much about what you eat. You can just enjoy your life. Well, only good carbs are recommended, and you should target lower carbs in your meal.

My potassium is low. What food is good for me?

I recommend that you take a potassium supplement instead of thinking of getting more potassium from food since in diabetes one of the treatments is to control your food intake. However, you might be able to incorporate the following food into your diet.

1. **Nuts:** Almonds,
2. **Fruit:** blackberries, apricots, avocados, dried apricots, bananas, dates, grapefruits, nectarines and oranges.
3. **Vegetables:** broccoli, Brussel sprouts, artichokes, acorn squash, spinach, mushrooms, carrots and tomatoes.
4. **Other:** sweet potatoes, coconut water, yogurt, white beans, beets, clams, lentils, okra, soymilk, salmon and tuna.

Chapter 11: Let's talk about sweeteners

What are the Sweeteners?

We know too much sugar is not a good thing. Now people are turning to sweeteners and think they are better alternatives. They may not be.

In the United States, six intensely sweet sugar substitutes have been approved for use. They are stevia, aspartame, sucralose, neotame, acesulfame potassium, and saccharin.

FDA and GRAS approved artificial sweeteners and brands			
Sweetener	Approval Date	Sweetness Factor (Relative to sugar)	Products
Saccharin	1958	200-700	Sweet'N Low, Sweet Twin, Sugar Twin
Aspartame	1981	200	NutraSweet, Equal
Acesulfame Potassium	1988	200	Sunnet, Sweet One
Sucralose	1998	600	Splenda
Neotame	2002	8000	Newtame
Advantame	2014	20,000	
Stevia/rebaudioside			Sweet Leaf, Sun Crystals, Stevia, Truvia, PureVia
Extracts from swingle fruit/monk fruit			

Is Aspartame marketed as NutraSweet toxic?

Lots of gums and sodas use this product. Aspartame is a methyl ester of the aspartic acid/phenylalanine dipeptide. Its metabolites are aspartate, phenylalanine and methanol.

Methanol is also called wood alcohol which is metabolized to formaldehyde. Formaldehyde is usually used to embalm a dead body or to keep a biopsy from decaying. It is a known poison to the central nervous system, and it may cause headaches, migraines, blindness, coma, and death. People say the amount of aspartame in soda is very, very low. The amount may be low, and it may be okay for some people, but not for me.

What do we know about sucralose?

Common brand names of sucralose-based sweeteners are Splenda, Sukrana, SucraPlus, Candys, Cukren and Nevella. Sucralose is a highly heat-stable artificial sweetener, allowing it to be used in many recipes with little or no sugar. However, in its pure state, sucralose begins to decompose into polychlorinated dibenzo-p-dioxins and other highly toxic substances at temperatures above 119 °C or 246 °F. Sucralose has been linked to leukemia, and reduced intestinal microflora which causes increased body weight, and increased levels of P-glycoprotein in rats.

What is neotame?

It is structured similar to aspartame. There is no production of phenylalanines, therefore it is safe for PKU patients. However, it also produces formaldehyde which has the same hazardous effect as aspartame.

What is acesulfame potassium?

Known as acesulfame K or ace K. K is the chemical symbol for potassium. Ace K is marketed under the trade names Sunett and Sweet One. In chemical structure acesulfame potassium is the potassium salt of 6-methyl-1,2,3-oxathiazine-4(3H)-one 2,2-dioxide. Studies in rodents show acesulfame might cause cancer and cognitive dysfunction.

What is saccharin?

Saccharin was discovered in 1879 when Constantin Fahlberg, a Johns Hopkins University scientist working on coal-tar derivatives, noticed a substance on his hands and arms that tasted sweet. It is now sold under brands such as Sweet 'N Low, Sweet Twin and Necta Sweet.

Studies in laboratory rats during the early 1970s linked saccharin with the development of bladder cancer in rodents.

What is Equal?

Equal is a brand of artificial sweetener containing aspartame, dextrose and maltodextrin.

What is stevia?

Stevia is a genus of about 240 species of herbs and shrubs in the sunflower family. These plants are native to subtropical and tropical regions from western North America to South America. The species Stevia Rebaudiana, commonly known as sweet leaf, sugar leaf, or simply stevia, is widely grown for its sweet leaves. In 1931, two French chemists isolated the glycosides that give stevia its sweet taste. These compounds, stevioside and rebaudioside A, are 250–300 times as sweet as sucrose and are heat-stable, pH-stable, and not fermentable.

Truvia is a consumer brand of stevia sweetener contains erythritol and rebiana, marketed by Coca Cola and Cargill.

PureVia is another brand of stevia marketed by Pepsico and Pure Circle.

SweetLeaf Is a stevia product by Wisdom Natural Brands

In its history, there has been lots of controversy about stevia's health effects. This includes the possibility it may be carcinogenic. However, it seems safe to say, that when consumed in reasonable amounts, stevia may be an exceptional natural plant-based sugar substitute.

Stevia is now present in a number of foods and beverages in the US, including Gatorade's G2, Vitaminwater Zero, SoBe Lifewater Zero, Crystal Light and Sprite Green.

Can I eat honey or use honey as sweetener?

Honey is actually simple sugar digested by bees. So, it is the same as sugar. I do not recommend using honey as a sweetener.

Chapter 12: Let's answer questions about holiday eating

Why do holidays always mess up my diabetes control?

This is a good question. Here are four reasons this could happen.

1. Holidays can put lots of extra stress on you. You might have been short of time for shopping, short of money for doing the things you want to do. You might be short of ideas for shopping or entertaining your family or friends. You know what? We always are short of something and this increases our stress. Not just shopping, you might be short of ideas for preparing a holiday party. Or, you might be short of time to go to all the parties. Or, you might worry that you have too many good ideas like asking this question. I guess I should say we always have a lot of things going on during the holidays that can cause us stress. Stress is not good for blood sugar control.

2. You might eat more. Food is always at the center of celebrations. We all focus too much on the food. The holiday food seems to always have too much added sugar, salt and fat. This is why we like our favorite foods. It is not easy to pass our favorite foods during the holidays.

3. You might drink some alcohol. Alcohol is part of the holidays for many people. Lots of people might not normally drink, but during the holidays, all sorts of alcoholic beverages are available, and they might be tempted to drink some.

4. You might move less. Holidays are most often the time when friends and family get together to catch up for the year. People sit, talk or play card games.

How can I lower my stress during the holidays?

Let's face it. Everyone has some stress no matter who you are. Look at the pictures of a president from year to year. You will see the stress is showing on his face, hair and body.

For me, here are three ways I use to reduce my stress. I believe that they can also work for you.

1. Identify where the stress is coming from. It is too much of something or too little of something. This is very important. If you do not know the cause, then you cannot really tackle it. Also, do not identify the wrong source. Sometimes, the source can be disguised. You need to dig deep and find the true source of the stress.

    A good idea is to list your sources of stress. This will give you a better picture of your situation. Even if you have many sources of stress, you might be overwhelmed already, but after you write them down, you will have a much clearer picture.

2. Ask yourself if this is something you can control, or is it something out of your control. If you can control it, do something about it. For example, if you can control the situation, then take measures to do something. If you cannot control the situation, try your best to let it go. Sometimes you can brainstorm and count the options. Then you might be able to do something about it.

3. Exercise. Exercise is not only good for diabetes, but it is also good for reducing your stress.

I am short of money for the holidays. Do you have any suggestions?

Taking care of diabetes is very expensive. Copays, deductibles, donut holes, you name it. As a doctor, I feel the pain every day for my patients. Many patients have to cut down their medicine to put food on the table. One time, I saw a patient at a hospital. He was admitted for something else, and in the chart I saw that he was taking over 300 units a day of insulin. However, when I sat down and talked to him, I learned that he had been taking it every other day and every other meal. He was not taking 300 units a day because it was so expensive, and he could not afford it. He did not want to tell his doctor because he was embarrassed. At his discharge, I was able to reduce him to 60 units every day. I have so many other similar stories to share.

Here are five suggestions I have to help you reduce your holiday financial stress:

1. Always let your doctor know if you cannot pay for a certain medication. Most of the time, we can find another alternative version which may be more affordable. Your doctor might have some coupons and samples to give you some relief.
2. Let your family and friends know that you are in financial trouble. They might have a charity budget. They might be able to help.
3. Reduce your holiday giving list. Honest to say, most gifts are useless anyway. You do not need to give everybody a gift. Even if they are expecting it, you do not have to give it. You can say you are sorry that you are not able to buy them a gift this year. Tell them you are stressed out financially, and that you need the money to buy medicine for diabetes.
4. Buy gifts while they are on sale. If there is someone you feel you have to give a gift to, you do not have to wait to the last minute. You can buy a gift after Christmas for next year's Christmas.
5. If you have talent, you can make a gift yourself. It will be much more valuable and more meaningful. Believe it or not, your gift receiver will appreciate it more since you put more thought into it, and you get a chance to show off your talent.

Holidays have so many parties and so much food. I cannot resist all the good food and it is only once a year. What can I do?

Here are some things to think about that may help you avoid those holiday food temptations:

1. You do not have to attend every party and put yourself into temptation and stress. These days, we are on lots of social media and we all know what is going on.
2. You do not have to try every food on the table. First, look at the table. Then, choose the one you really do not want to pass by.
3. Consider eating some salad or greens or cooked vegetables first. The fiber will slow down your digestion and slow down the increase in your sugar.
4. Be careful before you have some soup. Soups are usually broth based or cream based. Broth-based soups usually have high salt; cream-based soups have high calories. If your blood pressure is well controlled, it is reasonable to have some broth-based soup.
5. Try to save your stomach for the entree instead of the appetizer. Stay away from chips, crackers, cheese and high-calorie items.
6. Use portion control for entrees. Portion control is always important. If you have options, choose lean baked, broiled or grilled meat. Fish is more desirable if available. Stay away from starches, like potatoes (smashed or whole).
7. Dessert. Try to pass if you can. Otherwise, try very small slices.

I have type 1 diabetes and I am using an insulin pump. What can I do to control my holiday meals better?

The first thing you need to do is to prepare ahead of time. Before the holidays, talk to your doctor. Tell him or her your holiday specifics so specific recommendation can be made.

Here are five ideas that may help you control your sugar better during the holidays:

1. Now the FDA has approved a closed loop Medtronic insulin pump. I think a more competitive pump will be out soon. If you are already wearing such a pump, presumably, you do not need to worry too much. The pump will adjust your insulin automatically unless your eating exceeds the pump's maximal insulin delivery. You still need to announce your meal and gauge the carbs.
2. Since you ask this question, you most likely you do not have such a pump. If you have a CGM, you can give yourself a bolus every 2 hours, based on CGM data. The insulin pump will count the insulin onboard. The chance to develop hypoglycemia is low. Certainly, you need to be vigilant all the time. I assume you are using the bolus wizard.
3. If you are using an insulin pump without CGM, there are still many options you can try. Certainly none of them is completely hypo or hyperglycemia proof.
4. You can estimate how much you want to eat, and then you can use an extended or a combination bolus like dual wave, or square wave to cover your extended eating hours.
5. You can check in the middle of your eating, and give yourself a bolus. You can check at the end of your eating and give another bolus.

I am taking multiple daily injections of insulin to control my diabetes. What can I do for holiday eating?

If you are using multiple injections instead of insulin pump, you can estimate how much you are going to eat. Most of the time, you eat at least 30% or 100% more than usual. Based on your estimation, you can give more insulin before you eat. This can become very tricky. I recommend that you give more insulin in stages if you eat your holiday meals over a few hours. Again, check your sugar every 2 hours, and give half of your sliding scale every 2 hours if your sugar is persistently high. The reason to use half of the sliding scale is that this is a way to count the insulin that is already in your body that will still have an effect for at least 2 hours. This way you will prevent the stack effect which can lead to prolonged hypoglycemia.

A stack effect happens when you use more than one injection of fast acting insulin in less than 4 hours. If fast acting insulin is given every two hours, its effect overlaps the previously injected insulin. This is what the stack effect means. This could lower the sugar faster than expected and cause hypoglycemia.

I am using the basal insulin. Is there anything I can do for holiday eating?

If you are using a once a day long-acting insulin, it will be more challenging. On the day of the "big feast" you can try 25-50% more of basal insulin. If you are giving yourself insulin at night, you can give another 25%-50% of your regular basal insulin in the morning. Certainly again, do not forget to check your sugar.

I am taking oral medications. Anything can I do for holiday eating?

If you are not taking insulin, I do not recommend you take more medications.

For everyone, I recommend some moderate exercising before and after a big feast. Strenuous exercising is not recommended, especially after you eat a big meal.

Everyone is different. You need to learn your own body and make adjustments accordingly.

Chapter 13: Diabetes and exercise

For a normal person, what does short-term exercise do to our body sugar?

In a normal person, the muscles use glycogen as fuel for energy. A medium average 150-pound adult man has around 300 grams of sugar in the muscles which provide 1200 Kcal of energy. When the sugar in the blood stream begins to drop slightly, the liver glycogen begins to be mobilized. A 150 pound man has around 100 grams of glycogen in the liver. It can provide 400-500 kcal.

If the exercise continues, even before it uses up all the glycogen, lipolysis begins to release fatty acids and glycerol to be used for energy.

For a normal person, what does long-term exercise do to the body?

Long-term exercise makes the body use energy more efficiently. The sugar transporters are increased, the mitochondria (the place in our body's cells that produce energy) are increased. The muscles also become bigger and stronger.

Why is exercise important to diabetes?

Exercise and physical activity is good for everybody including diabetics. It makes insulin work better. It lowers your sugar by insulin dependent and independent pathways. It also lowers your blood pressure and cholesterol. It lowers your risk for heart disease and stroke. It helps you to lose weight and maintain your health. It increases your sense of wellbeing. It helps you sleep better. It helps to relieve your stress. It makes your heart and muscles stronger. It makes your bones stronger and less likely to break easily. It makes your joints more flexible. Exercise makes your balance better, and you are less likely to fall. It also helps to reduce symptoms of depression.

I have type 2 diabetes, and otherwise I am healthy and fit. Is there anything I need to do before I exercise?

If you have type 2 diabetes and no other complications, and if you are not using insulin or some medications like sulfonylureas, which can cause hypoglycemia, you do not have to take diabetes specific precautions. Follow the recommendations for people without diabetes.

If you are taking insulin or medications like sulfonylureas, you might need to reduce medications since exercise might cause hypoglycemia.

You also need to exercise with someone in case you develop hypoglycemia and you need to keep a "diabetes kit" with you. In the kit, you need to have a glucometer to check your sugar and some candy or something with sugar, which can raise your blood sugar quickly.

If you are taking SGLT2 antagonist like Invokana, Farxiga, or Jardiance or combinations, you need to take extra caution to avoid dehydration. Never exercise without taking water with you.

Can I drink Gatorade or another sport drink while I am exercising?

You certainly can. The issue is that if you are not doing strenuous exercise, you might not need a sport drink. Besides, all Gatorade and other sport drinks contain some sort of sugar, which might raise your sugar.

If you are doing very strenuous exercise like a marathon, then sport drinks might help you. You certainly need to monitor your sugar.

Is the G2 version better than regular Gatorade?

The G2 version has less sugar, 3% instead of the 6% which is in the regular version. If you are doing moderate exercise, and your sugar is not tending to drop in the middle of the exercise, or after the exercise, you can try the G2 version.

Do you recommend other sport drinks?

I think most of them are pretty much the same. They do have some difference in electrolytes contents and sugar content. You need to choose a sport drink based on how your body responds to it.

Here is a comparison of some of the popular sports drinks.

Product Serving Size 8 Oz. (240mL)	Total Calories	Total Carbs (g)	Sugar (g)	Sodium (mg)	Potassium (mg)
Accelerade	80	15	14	120	15
CamelBak Elixir	<5	<1	—	136	23
Cliff Shot Electrolyte	80	19	10	180-200	50
Cliff Quench	45	11	10	130	35
Cytomax	71	18	10	96	48
First Endurance EPS	63	16	11	180	107
Gatorade	50	14	14	110	30
Gatorade Endurance	50	14	14	200	90
Gatorade G2	25	7	7	110	30
GU Electrolyte Brew	50	13	4	125	20
GU_2O	<54	13	3	122	21
Heed	51	13	1	20	8
HYPR Sports Drink	71	19	—	151	—
Nuun	<5	<1	—	187	51
PowerADE	60	15	15	52	32
PowerADE Zero	0	0	0	100	250
Propel	10	2	2	75	0
CarboPro 2.6 Oz	200	50	0	150	100

I am using a wristband to monitor my activities. Is it accurate?

I saw one study that concluded if you are using a treadmill, it is quite accurate. If you are doing something like stroller pushing, it under counts your activity. The study also found that the devices were less accurate when worn on the person's dominant wrist.

Should I join a gym?

Studies show people tend to be more active when they join a gym. When you have a paid membership, you tend to exercise more. At the gym, you can also get consults from exercise professionals about what kind of exercise is good for you based on your fitness and physical condition.

I am too busy to do any exercise. What can I do?

Researchers found that short-burst exercise is as good as long and moderate exercise. If you are generally healthy, except for diabetes, you can try some so-called short-burst exercises. Be sure to include at least two minutes to warm up and three minutes to cool down. You can do two minutes of full-intensity exercise such as running or cycling.

When is it better to exercise, before a meal or after a meal?

Studies have found that if you exercise after a meal, your need for insulin will be reduced. When you exercise before a meal, your insulin sensitivity will increase after the meal. If you are taking insulin, you can reduce your insulin use. If you are taking a sulfonylurea medication, you can reduce it also.

My recommendation is that if you are on insulin and your sugar is under perfect control, and if you start walking before or after the meal, you can reduce your insulin by 20% to start with. Based on your response, you can adjust your premeal insulin.

Is it better to exercise after a meal so I will not have hypoglycemia?

It is true your chances of having hypoglycemia are reduced if you exercise after a meal. I do not recommend for you to do strenuous exercise immediately after a meal. However, it is okay to start walking 10-15 minutes after a meal.

I do not have time during the day. Can I do my exercise at night?

This is a difficult question. Exercise has different effects on different people. For most people exercise will increase their alertness due to the secretion of adrenaline and cortisol. These hormones might affect your sleep. If you want to do exercise at night, I recommend you do it two hours before you go to bed. This will minimize the unfavorable effect on your sleep.

What kind of exercise is good for diabetes?

All kinds of physical activities are good for diabetes. Based on ADA research, the two most important types of exercise for diabetes are aerobic exercise and strength (resistance) training.

What is aerobic exercise?

Aerobic simply means that your cardiovascular system can supply enough oxygen to the muscles for energy. In the gym, it is known as cardio.

Examples of aerobic exercises are:

- cardio machines
- swimming
- hiking
- dancing
- cycling / running
- walking
- kickboxing
- cross country skiing

However, when you perform an exercise at an intensity which exceeds your heart and lung capacity to supply enough oxygen to your muscles, then the aerobic exercise becomes an anaerobic exercise.

What is resistance training?

Resistance (strength) training is using weights to train your muscles.

Examples of resistance training are:

1. Using your own body weight--like pushups, pull-ups, abdominal crunches and leg squats.
2. Using free weights, like barbells and dumbbells.
3. Using weight machines. There are many different weight machines you can use if you go to a gym or fitness center. You certainly can also buy a weight machine.
4. Using resistance bands. They come in different strengths and colors. They all are very affordable. You can use them almost anywhere.

I have a history of cardiovascular disease. What should I pay more attention to while exercising?

Here are seven things to pay attention to while exercising:

1. Start slow and increase intensity slowly.
2. Stop if you have chest pain, shortness of breath, or other discomfort. See your cardiologist.
3. Do not get dehydrated.
4. Do not do strenuous exercise under the sun.
5. Do not do exercise under extreme weather conditions.
6. You can do resistance exercises, with low weights and moderate intensity. Do not exceed your capacity.
7. Ideally, get an exercise prescription for a physical therapist.

I have retinopathy. What should I pay more attention to while I exercise?

There are actually different kinds of retinopathy. If you have diabetic proliferation retinopathy, you certainly should not do strenuous exercise or resistance training, since in proliferative retinopathy, the new fragile cells developed on the optic disc. Too much pressure can cause leakage or hemorrhaging into the eye resulting in loss of vision. You may also be at risk for retina detachment.

Therefore, it is recommended that you start slow and go slowly with low to moderate intensity. This includes activities like slow biking, walking, ballroom dancing, and other low-impact activities. Do not do anything with movement that causes you to lower your head or hold your breath.

I have neuropathy. What should I remember when I do my exercise?

Mild neuropathy does not affect your balance, but severe neuropathy does. If you feel unstable, you need to choose exercises that will not cause you to fall.

If your neuropathy does not affect your walking or jogging, it is okay to continue. If your neuropathy is so severe that you are not balanced, you should not walk as an exercise. If you can swim, it is a great exercise. Stationary biking is safe for patients with neuropathy.

 Examine your feet before you start exercising and after you finish to make sure you do not have any cuts or ulcers.

I have Charcot foot. What can I do for exercise?

This bad form of neuropathy most often occurs with type 1 diabetes. The foot bones are repeatedly fractured and this causes deformation.

You should not walk as an exercise. You certainly should not jog or run. Walking in the pool may be okay depending on your severity. The idea is that you should stay off your feet as long as possible. You should also have diabetic shoes that have a good fit and great support.

Arm biking can be a good form of exercise. Floor exercises are good, too.

If you have access to a pool, swimming will be the best exercise for you. If you do not know how to swim, you can learn or just walk in the pool.

You should not do water exercise if you have an open wound. As a rule of thumb, you should avoid putting weight on your foot when you exercise.

You should exercise with someone else since you most likely have type 1 diabetes which is prone to cause hypoglycemia.

I have nephropathy. What should I pay attention to during exercise?

Strenuous exercise increases your blood pressure and increases your blood pressure to the kidneys. This can increase the protein in the urine and might worsen your nephropathy. Therefore, you should not do strenuous exercise. Chinese Tai Chi is good. Swimming (water aerobics), cycling and Yoga are good, too.

How should I work with a personal trainer?

If you are lucky enough and able to hire a personal trainer, here are some recommendations:

1. If possible, get a recommendation from your friends who have used the personal trainer before.
2. Check credentials. Your trainer might be certified under ACSM (American College of Sports Medicine); NASM (National Academy of Sports Medicine); NSCA (National Strength and Conditioning Association).
3. Ask your trainer some questions to get to know them better. You can ask about his or her previous experience working with diabetics and other specific conditions you might have. It

is very important to know if he or she has some basic knowledge of diabetes.
4. Write down the list of conditions you have and communicate this to your personal trainer. This is very important. Since certain conditions mean you need to stay away from certain types of exercise. For example, if you have retinopathy, you should not do any exercise to increase the pressure to your retina. If you are not very clear about your condition, you can ask your doctor to help you.
5. Educate your trainer. Let your trainer know how to observe hypo or hyperglycemia, and discuss plans to handle problems beforehand.
6. If you have a CGM and insulin pump, educate your trainer about what it can do and what it cannot do.

Chapter 14: Diabetes and travel

Why should I have a travel plan for my diabetes?

For the best diabetes control, you need to have a scheduled life, but travel breaks every routine you might have. When you travel, things change like your food, your activities, your sleep, even your time zone. Travel can present significant challenges to your diabetes control. If you are mindful and prepared, I am sure it will pay off, and you will enjoy your travel and vacation much more.

What and how should I prepare for my travel?

As we already discussed, there are some general rules, and some specifics you need to consider. Your travel preparations depend on what kind of diabetes you have, what regimen you are on and how you will be traveling. There are many specifics, and we cannot know every scenario, but we will discuss some specifics in the questions that follow.

I have type 1 diabetes and I am using an insulin pump, how should I prepare for travel? Do you have a checklist?

Yes, I do. Here is the checklist for you.

- ✓ Bring your pump. This is obvious.
- ✓ Travel bag.
- ✓ Insulin. Take more than you estimate you might need.
- ✓ Infusion sets. Take more than you need.
- ✓ Batteries. Take extra batteries in the right sizes.
- ✓ Glucometer, strips, lancets and alcohol swipes.
- ✓ Ketostix
- ✓ Your insulin pump failure supplies like insulin pen, needles or syringes
- ✓ Always wear you diabetes alert bracelet.

- ✓ Hypoglycemia kit. Snacks for mild hypoglycemia and your glucagon emergency kit.
- ✓ Do not forget other medications for other conditions.
- ✓ Some antibiotics for UTI or yeast infection if you think you need them.
- ✓ Do not forget your doctor's office telephone number and your pump manufacturer's representative number.

I have type 1 diabetes and I am on basal and bolus regimen. How should I prepare for travel? Do you have a checklist?

Here is a checklist for you:

- ✓ Your insulins both-long-acting and short-acting.
- ✓ Glucometer, strips and lancets and alcohol swipes.
- ✓ Hypoglycemia kit with snacks for mild hypoglycemia and a glucagon emergency kit.
- ✓ Ketostix.
- ✓ Diabetic alert bracelet.
- ✓ Do not forget other medications for other conditions.
- ✓ Some antibiotics for UTI or yeast infection if you think you need them.
- ✓ Do not forget your doctor's office telephone number.
- ✓ Travel bag.
- ✓ Sharps disposal container or similar hard surface disposal container.

I have type 2 diabetes and I am taking insulin. What should I do to prepare for travel?

You should use the checklist above for type 1 diabetes basal and bolus regimen.

I am traveling by plane. Any TSA tips?

Here are some TSA tips for you.

1. Make sure you bring all your medications in carry-ons.
2. Put all the insulin vials and pens in a bag and declare them.
3. You do not need a letter from your doctor to bring diabetes supplies onto a plane. If you want one, you can always ask for one from your doctor's office.
4. If you wear an insulin pump, the pump manufacturer usually advises against it being screened by imaging technology. Technically speaking, there should be no problem for it to be screened by an x-ray or a metal detector. I have patients who say they let their pump go through the x-ray machine. If you don't want to do this, you can let the TSA do a pat down check, then they will usually check for explosive residues.
5. If you wear a sensor, you are advised not to use the whole body scanner. I do not know of any research, but the manufacturer usually advises against it.
6. If you have further questions or concerns, you can call TSA toll free 855-782-2227.

I have type 1 diabetes, and I am on an insulin pump. I will fly over a few time zones. How do I change my pump settings?

First, as we discussed, you should know your basal rates. Some patients have one single basal rate. Some patients have multiple basal rates and have significant changes. Again, you should be mindful that your basal rate needs changing if your lifestyle changes. Travel changes your lifestyle. Checking your sugar is the key.

Here is a way you can test to see if your basal rate has not changed too much when you get up and when you go to sleep. You can simply keep the same setting and switch to the local time when you get there. You can try the average basal rate as your temporary rate (=total basal units/24), if you have a variable basal rate.

You can also visit your doctor's office. Discuss possible lifestyle changes, and your doctor can set up a second basal rate for you. When you get to the new time zone, you can change the time and restart the basal.

Travel sometimes can be unpredictable. Ask your doctor to recommend a single basal rate based on your proposed activities. Do this if you would like to have a relatively conservative basal rate, and then if your sugar is too high, you can compensate with bolus. Therefore, checking your sugar is the key. Bring more strips and lancets to monitor your sugar since you might test many more times than usual.

I am on long-acting and short-acting insulin. I will fly east over a few time zones. What should I do?

If you fly east, the day of flying will be shorter. If the time change is just under 4 hours difference, you might just reduce your basal by 10-20%, or no change at all if your sugar has not been well-controlled. When you reach your destination, change your watch to the local time and continue your regular basal. You should continue your same bolus dosage, using the insulin carbohydrate ratio and sliding scale (correction).

If you fly east and the time change is 4-8 hours, you can reduce your basal insulin by 30% on the day of flying.

If you fly east and the time zone change is over 8 hours, you can reduce your basal insulin by 50%. If you give yourself basal every 12 hours, you can simply miss one dose.

I am on long-acting and short-acting insulin. I will fly west over a few time zones. What should I do to my basal insulin?

If you fly west, the day of flying will be longer. Again, if the time change is less than 8 hours, you might not need to make any changes to your basal insulin. You might just check your sugar 1-2 more times and give some correction if needed.

If you fly west and the time change is 8 hours or more, I recommend you keep your original time zone on the airplane, and give the basal insulin at the usual time. When you get to your destination, you can miss one dose, just use the correction or sliding scale every 4 hours, until the next usual basal dose based on the new destination time. However, if you are using the basal every 12 hours, then you can switch to local time without too much difficulty. You do not need to miss any doses.

I am on oral diabetes medications. What should I do if I travel over a few time zones?

There are a few oral medication categories.

If you are taking sulfonylurea and traveling east, you might want to reduce the dose in the day of travel, or after adjusting to the local time. If you travel to the west and the time difference is less than 8 hours, you can adjust to the local time after your arrival.

If you are taking medications like glinides, you can continue to take it with meals.

If you are taking other medications, you can follow the instructions for sulfonylurea.

If you are taking daily injections like Victoza, it is okay to continue the current regimen with no change. Or, you can miss one dose based on which way you are traveling.

If you are taking a once a week injection, then you really do not need to worry. After arriving in the new time zone, you can continue your regimen.

Chapter 15: How should I prepare for a colonoscopy or outpatient surgery?

What should I do when I am preparing for a colonoscopy?

Colonoscopy is a common procedure that most patients will have at least once in their lifetime. The day before the procedure, you will prepare for the procedure by taking a clear liquid diet and some laxatives.

Diabetes control relies on diet, while medication is adjusted based on your diet. Because your diet is being changed drastically for the procedure, your diabetes medication will also need to be adjusted. Here are some suggestions but you will need to go through these with your gastroenterologist and the doctor who is taking care of your diabetes.

Your diet will be clear liquids.

The following drinks are recommended:

- water (plain, carbonated or fruit flavor)
- fruit juices without pulp, such as apple, or white grape (not red grape juice)
- sodas are fine
- gelatin (no red color)
- tea or coffee without cream or milk
- strained tomato or vegetable juice (not smoothies)
- sport drinks like Gatorade
- clear, fat-free broth (bouillon or consommé-you can buy or make yourself)
- ice pops without milk, bits of fruits

Your medication also depends on how many carbs (sugar) you are drinking. Generally speaking:

- If you have type 2 diabetes and are on oral medications–take half of your medication the day before and do not take any oral medication on the day of the procedure. If you finish the

procedure very early in the morning, and resume your diet, you can resume your oral medication.
- If you have type 2 diabetes and are only on metformin, it is okay not to take metformin the day before and on the day you have procedure.
- If you have type 2 diabetes and are on long-acting insulin, you can take half the dose you are taking the day before and on the day of procedure if you have reasonably good control before the procedure. However, if your blood sugar has been over 200, you can continue your usual dose.
- Certainly you need to check your sugar at least 4 times a day, every 4-6 hours and anytime you feel your sugar may be low.
- If you are taking multiple shots, to be safe, I recommend you take ⅓ to half of your dose before each meal(your liquid meal) of the fast-acting and take half of the long-acting. You can continue to use the sliding scale.
- However, if you have type 1 diabetes and you are on an insulin pump, I recommend that you use the half dose on the sliding scale at bedtime. If your blood sugar is reasonably controlled, then you should be able to continue to use your pump the day before. Some gastroenterologists do not feel comfortable allowing you to keep the insulin pump on. If this is the case, it is okay for you to take it off, because most colonoscopies only last 30-60 minutes. However, if you are having a more complicated procedure that you expect to be longer, you need to be on an insulin pump or substitute with basal long-acting insulin.
- If you have type 1 diabetes and you are on multiple shots daily, certainly, you do not need premeal insulin on the day of the procedure since you are not eating. You need to continue the basal insulin and the sliding scale. If you are drinking anything with carbs, you need to give insulin depending on your carb ratio. If you do not know your carb ratio and cannot reach your doctor,

you can try to give a third of your fixed dose pre-meal insulin for every cup of sugary drink.

What should I do if I am going to have surgery tomorrow?

For hospitalized surgery, your surgeon or other health care personnel will decide what to do. In the case of outpatient surgery and your surgeon does not give you instructions, here are your guidelines. Following your surgeon's instructions is very important. These recommendations are not meant to replace your surgeon's recommendations.

This also depends on what type of diabetes, what kind of surgery, and how long your surgery lasts.

1. If you have type 2 diabetes and are on oral medications, if your surgery is minor and your surgeon does not ask you to fast, you can continue your same regimen.
2. If you have type 2 diabetes and are on oral medications, if your surgeon asks you to fast overnight, the second day you can omit the oral diabetes medication. Your surgery team will give you insulin if your sugar is too high.
3. If you have type 2 diabetes and you have gastroparesis, you might want to fast longer than overnight if fasting is required for your surgery.
4. If you have type 2 diabetes and you are on basal insulin, and if your sugar has been well-controlled with no significant lows or highs, no matter what kind of surgery, you can continue the same dose of long-acting basal insulin. If you have had frequent low sugar before, I recommend you to use half of your basal insulin.
5. If you have type 2 diabetes and you are on multiple shots involving long-acting and short-acting insulin, you can keep the same dose of basal insulin, and stop the short-acting dose. However, if you have some low sugar episodes before the

surgery, I recommend you to cut down your basal insulin by half.

6. If you have type 1 diabetes, and you are on an insulin pump, and you do not have frequent lows, I recommend keeping the insulin pump on if possible.

7. If your procedure is under 1 hour, it is okay to be off your insulin pump if your surgeon requests. If you expect your procedure to be longer or other things happen, you need to be on basal insulin or fast-acting insulin. Your surgeon should know how to take care of it.

8. If you have type 1 diabetes and you are on basal and bolus regimen, and you do not have significant lows, you can continue to take the same dose of basal insulin. If you have frequent lows, I recommend you to reduce your basal insulin by half.

9. If you have type 1 diabetes and you are on premix insulin, it can be very challenging. If your surgery is less than 8 hours after your last dose and the surgery is very short, it is okay to miss one dose. If your surgery is longer than 8 hours after your last insulin dose, you need to give yourself some insulin. Discuss this with your doctor beforehand. I recommend you have surgery early in the day so you do not have to fast very long. If you do not have insulin for longer than 12 hours, you might develop DKA (diabetic ketoacidosis).

Chapter 16: 10 questions about vaccinations

Why should I get vaccinated?

Diabetes is associated with a 6-fold increase in hospitalization and a 3-fold increase in death from complications of influenza or pneumonia. Diabetes patients also double their risk for hepatitis B.

When should I get a pneumonia shot?

The ADA (American Diabetes Association) recommends to give pneumonia shots to all diabetics 2 years old and older.

What forms of pneumonia shots do we have?

We have PCV13 and PPSV23. PCV -(pneumococcal conjugate vaccine) 13 has 13 serotypes of pneumococcus. These 13 types account for the majority of invasive pneumococcal disease (IPD) in the US, including serotype 19A, which is the most common IPD-causing serotype in young children. Pneumococcal polysaccharide vaccine (PPSV23) contains the same 12 serotypes in PCV13 and 11 more than PCV13.

What pneumonia shot should I get?

If you are younger than 65, you only need PPSV23, one shot is enough. If you are older than 65, you need to get both PCV13 and PPSV23. First you get one dose of PPSV23, but should be 5 years after the previous dose if you had PPSV23 before. Then one dose of PCV13 which should be at least 1 year after. PPSV23 should be given every 5 years.

How often should I get an influenza (flu) shot?

Even the general public it is recommended to have a flu shot every year. You should, too.

Should I get a stronger flu shot?

This is not necessary.

Why should I get Hepatitis B shot?

It is found that diabetes has higher risk for hepatitis B. The reason is not clear. One thing is for sure, diabetics go to health care facilities more often which increases their risk.

How often should I get Hepatitis B vaccine?

Hepatitis B vaccine is a series of three shots. The second shot should be one month later, and the last shot should be six months later. Usually you only need one series of shots in your lifetime. The effectiveness can be checked by an antibody titer.

When should I get shingles vaccine?

If you are 60 or older, you should get one dose of shingles vaccine. The vaccine is not recommended for people younger than 60, and it is only given once in a lifetime. The vaccine can only provide 50% protection and usually only lasts five years.

Should I get Tdap vaccine also?

It is not clear if diabetes patients have higher risk for tetanus, diphtheria, and pertussis. The vaccination should follow the recommendations for the general public. A Td booster should be given every 10 years. Substitute Tdap for Td once.

Chapter 17: Let's talk more about insulin pump failure.

Why do I need to be prepared for insulin pump failure?

An insulin pump is a delicate computerized insulin delivery device. This device is like any other device, and it can fail. The failure rate is different based on different pumps. There can be drive failures, software failures and battery failures. However, a kinked cannula is very commonly interpreted as a pump failure. The easiest fix is to change the infusion set. If you are on Omni-pod, the pod failure is also very common. You need to change the pod first to see if you can correct it.

How should I be prepared for an insulin pump failure?

Here are four things you can do to prepare for an insulin pump failure:

1. You need to have some troubleshooting skills for insulin pump failure.
2. Know your settings, like basal rate, carbohydrate ratio, and correction rate. Write them down. Keep them updated if changed, and keep them handy.
3. Have your pump manufacturer's telephone number handy. You might need it often.
4. Always, have extra bottles of insulin and syringes and other supplies you may need.

What to do if I think my pump fails?

If you are prepared, depending what you have, you have these options.

1. You should know your average total dose (basal + bolus), if you do not know this, think back how you used your last bottle of insulin, how many days did you take to finish it. For example, if you take 10 days to finish one bottle of 10 ml insulin (1,000 units), then your daily use is 100 units, but usually you can add 20% to waste.

Therefore, you are using 80 units every day. If you still can view the data in the pump, then you can check this information in the pump.

2. Then you can give your basal every 4 hours. For example, if your basal is 24 units, then 24 divided by 6 equals 4. You give 4 units of your fast insulin every 4 hours.
3. You will continue to use the same carb ratio for diet.
4. You can continue the same sensitivity for high sugar.
5. If you know the exact basal rate, you can use that basal rate every 2 hours. For example, if from 9am to 11 am, you have a basal rate of 1 unit per hour, then you can give 2 units at 9 am.
6. If you have Lantus or Levemir at home, and if it will be a few days before you can get your pump back, you might switch back to basal and bolus regimen which you were using before the pump.

    - If you know your basal rate, add together every 12 hours or every 24 hours of basal, and you can use Lantus every 12 hours or every 24 hours, and use Levemir every 12 hours.
    - Continue to use your usual carbohydrate ratio for meals and snacks. Use the sliding scale (correction) for high sugar.
    - Now we have more basal insulins to be used as once daily insulins. Tresiba takes 3-4 days to reach the steady state which might not be optimal for this situation. Toujeo also needs a few days to get the steady state, which is not ideal either. The new biosimilar Basaglar is presumably appropriate to use.

7. Contact your pump manufacturer representative and doctor's office if you need further help.

How should I take care of my insertion site?

It is crucial to choose a good site for the insulin pump insertion. The cannula is a foreign object which can induce an immune reaction which can cause inflammation, lipodystrophy and scar formation. The risks for repeated insertion at the same place, or leaving it in for too long, are too traumatic. Certainly, infection is the worst.

Here are six recommendations:

1. Always choose a smooth, fresh site (not used recently)
2. Choose the site at least 5 cm away from the previous site.
3. Ideally, do not to use the same site in the same month. Rotate the sites. For example, every month; you need to have 10 sites. Mark your sites into 10 regions. Rotate them in such a way that you only use one region once a month. Even in the same region, try to use as many different sites as possible. Remember, repeated injury can cause scars even for a very small injury.
4. Change your infusion set every three days. Try not to extend it to avoid the trouble of changing it or to save money. As I said, your body looks at the cannula like a foreign object, and it will cause inflammation. The inflammatory cells and fibers might block the cannula and cause less insulin to be delivered than intended.
5. If you see blood, you need to change your site.
6. If you have too much pain, something may be wrong. You need to change your site.

My sugar is high and I have ketones. What should I do?

Here are three things you need to know if you have high ketones:

1. If you have a fever, chest pain, nausea or vomiting, then you have to go to the ER.

2. If you think you are sick enough to go to the ER, then most likely you need to go.

3. However, if you still want to try to help yourself. Here are a few things you can do: drink lots of water, do not exercise, give yourself subcutaneous insulin and change the insertion site. As we already discussed you might have a cannula kinked.

My sugar is high but I do not have high ketones. What should I do?

It is very common for type 1 diabetics to have a high fluctuation of sugar, even for your sugar to go beyond to 500 or higher.

Here are six things you can do:

1. Think to see if you can find the reason you have high sugar. Did you eat something you should not have eaten like pizza? Did you forget to give a bolus, or are you on steroids? Or, do you have lots of pain or stress?

2. You can try to change the infusion sets.

3. Check your sugar and ketones every hour. It is okay to manage yourself by giving a correction scale of insulin if you continue to feel well.

4. Drink water, and give yourself another bolus-if the first bolus does not get your sugar down. Try to double the calculated bolus. Remember to let your family know what you are doing and monitor your sugar closely. They can help you monitor as well. Also, remember the stacking effect of insulin, which might get your sugar too low.

5. Do not go to bed until your sugar is stabilized.

6. Do not feel bad about going to the ER. Type 1 diabetes is a serious disease. Doctors and nurses take caring for you seriously.

What are the most common causes for high sugar experienced by your insulin pump patients?

1. Insertion site problems like the cannula was kinked or inserted into a scar.

2. The insulin was exposed to heat. After you changed your infusion set, and you are still not able to get your sugar down, you might need to change your insulin to a new batch.

3. A pod failure. The Omni-pod has a very high rate of failure.

Chapter 18: Diabetes and cholesterol

What are lipids?

Lipids are fats. They are groups of waxy like substances that are partly absorbed from the intestines and partly made in our bodies. Fat is not soluble in blood, therefore it is carried by a group of proteins called lipoproteins.

Why is it important to control lipids in diabetes?

The leading causes for morbidity and mortality are cardiovascular diseases including stroke, TIA, heart attack, and peripheral vascular disease. The risk for heart attack is doubled in diabetics. Controlling the lipids in diabetics is extremely important in controlling the risks.

What items are in the routine lipid profile test?

There are three things on the routine lipid profile:

1. Low-density-lipoprotein cholesterol (LDL-C), is usually called "bad cholesterol". Its main physiologic function is to deliver the cholesterol to the tissues where it is used. For example, cholesterol is used to make hormones like cortisol, estrogen, testosterone. A high LDL-C level is associated with a higher risk for cardiovascular diseases.

2. High-density-lipoprotein cholesterol (HDL-C), is usually called "good cholesterol". The main function for HDL is to deliver the excessive cholesterol back to the liver to be metabolized and eliminated from the body. Higher HDL levels are associated with a lower risk for cardiovascular diseases.

3. Triglycerides are the most common type of fat in the body. If your triglycerides are very high, you can see your blood become creamy like milk. The connection with cardiovascular disease has not been fully established. However, when the level is too high, it can cause pancreatitis and skin rashes.

What kind of lipid profile do we see in diabetes patients?

Typically, in diabetes the lipids are going in the wrong direction. The "good cholesterol" HDL is decreased to 30s, and the "bad cholesterol" LDL is increased and over 130, and the triglycerides are in the 200s.

Why do the triglyceride numbers change a lot from tests at different times?

Triglycerides are the most common fat. If you eat something with fat, it will show up in the blood right away. The number changes drastically based on what you eat. If you are checking after fasting, then the variation will be smaller.

Do we have a target to control our lipids?

In practice, I also consider recommendations from ADA (American Diabetes Association), AACE (American Association of Clinical Endocrinologists), ACC/AHA(American College of Cardiology/American Heart Association)

I use my own five guidelines:

1. For a diabetic patient who is not pregnant or not planning on becoming pregnant, I advise anyone at any age to get LDL down below 100.
2. For a diabetic patient who has a family history of cardiovascular disease (CAD) plus an LDL>130, I would try my test to get his or her LDL down below 100.
3. For patients who already have a history of cardiovascular disease (CAD), then the LDL target is below 70.
4. Strive to get HDL over 40.
5. Make sure to get triglycerides below 500, and try to get them below 150 if possible. However, if they are already below 500, I usually do not recommend medications.

Do I need to have a fasting lab test or not?

I usually do not recommend fasting for patients. As I discussed before, the LDL does not change much for most people when fasting or not fasting. Fasting has a lot of potential side effects such as severe low sugar. Since some of my patients live so far away, fasting also breaks their routine of taking drugs. I have patients who have not taken blood pressure medications and this leads to increased blood pressure. So, they should just come as if it was any other usual day of life. They should take all their medications and eat their usual breakfast.

I have a history of statin intolerance. Can I use statins again?

Around 10-25% of patients cannot tolerate statins due to muscle symptoms. However, experts say most of these patients do not have real statin intolerance. They found in a clinical trial that they had the same muscle pain even on a placebo.

Sometimes, the statin intolerance is also caused by drug interactions.

What do you recommend for statin intolerant patients?

Here are my top 12 recommendations for my statin intolerant patients:

1. Ask your doctor to review your medication list. Statins are one of the medications that are prone to have adverse interaction with other drugs.
2. Ask your doctor to check if you have untreated hypothyroidism.
3. Do not drink alcoholic beverages excessively.
4. Do not drink grapefruit juice. As a matter of fact, do not drink any kind of fruit juice.
5. You might consider reducing the dose, frequency, or changing to another statin.
6. For Asians in advanced age with poor liver and/or kidney function, your dose might need to be reduced.

7. Choose a different statin; if you used lipophilic statins like atorvastatin, fluvastatin, lovastatin and simvastatin before, you can try hydrophilic statins like pravastatin, pitavastatin, and rosuvastatin.
8. You can try Zetia which blocks the absorption of cholesterol.
9. You can try other bile sequestrans.
10. You can try plant sterols and stanols.
11. Some people use Chinese red yeast rice and have some good results. Red yeast rice is made from fermented rice which contains an active ingredient called monacolin K, which is structurally similar to lovastatin. The side effect is not really clear.
12. If you are qualified and your insurance pays for it, a new class of cholesterol medications, PCSK-9 inhibitors like Repatha and Praluent, can be considered.

What are other potential side effects of statins?

Besides the most common muscle side effects, statins might cause elevated liver enzymes or new onset of diabetes. Some unconfirmed claims are cancer, cognitive decline, lung disease, erectile dysfunction, cataracts, rheumatoid arthritis, gastrointestinal upset, lower extremity cramping, permanent liver or kidney damage.

Do statins really cause diabetes or make diabetes worse?

In some clinical trials, the group taking statins has increased risk for developing new onset of diabetes. In the study PROSPER (Prospective Study of Pravastatin in the Elderly at Risk) increased the risk for developing diabetes as high as 32%.

In other trials, other statins like atorvastatin in CARDS (Collaborative Atorvastatin Diabetes Study) and Crestor (rosuvastatin) in the JUPITER study (Justification for the Use of Statins in Primary Prevention: An Intervention Trial Evaluating Rosuvastatin) also showed to increase the risk for diabetes.

Statins also have been shown to increase A1c.

Why do statins cause diabetes?

We still do not know for sure why statins cause diabetes. Some research suggested that statins cause beta cell dysfunction and increase muscle insulin resistance.

Should I stop statins?

No, you should not.

The benefit of taking statins far outweighs the risk of new onset of diabetes and increased A1c.

Is there anything I can do to reduce the effect of statins on my diabetes?

Exercise is the best way. Exercise increases your insulin sensitivity. Statins reduce your insulin sensitivity.

Your doctor also uses some other medications to combat this phenomenon. Some research has shown that adding the bile acid Sequestrant Colesevelam is very useful. Colesevelam not only decreases your cholesterol further, but it also decreases your A1c.

Some patients also take Coenzymes Q10. This has not been proven in clinical trials, but there is no downside to taking it.

Is it useful to take Coenzyme Q10 to alleviate the side effects of statins?

Coenzyme Q10 is very important in metabolism. It is required for your body to produce ATP. It is also important as an antioxidant in cell membranes and lipoproteins.

Coenzyme Q10 is produced by our own body in the same pathway as cholesterol synthesis. Fortunately, coenzyme Q10 is also absorbed from food. The use of statins has not shown to have reduced coenzyme Q10 in most studies. There is one report that the level of Q10 was reduced. The use of coenzyme Q10 has not been shown to reduce the possible side effects of statins.

However, if you think this might help you, you can use them. The use of coenzyme Q10 does not have severe side effects. You can use the supplement safely as long as you buy it from a reputable source.

I have diabetes and renal failure. Should I be on statins?

Well, renal failure is a very broad term. It is classified into stages 1-5. Renal failure was classified as a cardiovascular disease equivalent by some lipid specialists, therefore statins are recommended for most patients. However, there are some specifics you might need to discuss with your doctor.

I have diabetes and renal failure. Which statins should I use?

Usually, I start with a low dose of any medication to see how you respond to it. If your eGFR (measures kidney function) is less than 30, usually I would not recommend more than the following doses:

- atorvastatin 20 mg
- rosuvastatin 10 mg
- simvastatin 40 mg
- pravastatin 40 mg
- fluvastatin 80 mg
- pitavastatin 2 mg

However, most patients with an eGFR less than 30, who are on high doses of statins, tolerate atorvastatin very well.

I am on hemodialysis. Should I stay on statins?

Based on some clinical trials including 4D (Die Deutsche Diabetes Dialyse), AURORA (A Study to Evaluate the Use of Rosuvastatin in Subjects on Regular Hemodialysis), and sub-group analysis of SHARP (Study of Heart and Renal Protection), the use of statins does not provide any benefit to patients on dialysis. Therefore, if you are on hemodialysis, statins are not recommended. However, if you have been on one already, and if you do not have any side effects, it is recommended that you continue it.

I have a renal transplant. Do you have any recommendations?

KDIGO (Kidney Disease Improving Global Outcomes) recommends treating all adult kidney transplant recipients with a statin, regardless of age. This recommendation is based mainly on the ALERT (Assessment of Lescol in Renal Transplantation) trial, which randomized 2102 renal transplant patients aged 30-75 with baseline total cholesterol 156– 251 mg/dl to fluvastatin 40 mg/day or placebo. The analysis found that the initiation of statin therapy early after the transplantation provided more benefit than that observed with late initiation.

Should I use Zetia?

A clinical study called SHARP was designed to study the use of Zetia on top of simvastatin on a wide range of renal function. It was found that the combination of simvastatin 20 mg plus Zetia 10 mg daily safely reduced the incidence of major atherosclerotic events.

Therefore, if your insurance pays for it, it is okay to use it.

What age should I start cholesterol treatment?

Now, many organizations including ACC/AHA (American College of Cardiology/American Heart Association) recommend the start of cholesterol treatment between the ages of 40-75. I consider this really mechanical and absurd. I practice medicine using both common sense and evidence-based medicine.

Atherosclerotic cardiovascular disease does not occur overnight or at a certain age, instead it is an accumulative event. If you have smoked for a long time, have had high cholesterol for a long time, or have had high sugar for a long time, this will increase your risk for cardiovascular disease. Evidence has also been found that atherosclerotic plaque starts to build up in the teenage years or earlier.

I try to keep everyone's LDL below 100 mg/dl. However if you are a female and have a risk for pregnancy, I will wait to start statins since statins affect fetal development. You want to take the least medication as possible while you are pregnant.

I want to know my cardiovascular risk. Do you know any tools I can use to calculate my risk?

As I said before, if you have diabetes you have high risk already. The risk is just risk. You need to keep unnecessary risk as low as possible. I usually do not calculate these risks. There are many tools from different risk calculators you can use from various databases.

Here are six online tools that can help you know your cardiovascular risk:

1. Framingham: http://cvdrisk.nhibi.nih.gov
2. Reynolds: reynoldsrikscore.org
3. MESA: mesa-nhibi.org
4. UKPDS:; dtu.ox.ac.uk/riskengine
5. Steno T1 risk engine: steno.shinyapps.io/T1RiskEngine/
6. Pooled Cohort Risk Assessment Equations: my.americanheart.org/cvriskcalculator

I have a renal transplant and I am on cyclosporine. What is the recommendation for statin choices?

Cyclosporine has many drug interactions with statins and other medications. The recommended statins and doses are fluvastatin 40 mg daily, atorvastatin 10 mg daily, rosuvastatin 5 mg daily, pravastatin 20 mg daily and simvastatin 20 mg daily.

Shunzhong Shawn Bao, M.D.

I have a renal transplant and I am not taking cyclosporine. Do I have to restrict the dose of statins?

Yes, you still have restrictions. Here are the dose recommendations: fluvastatin 80 mg daily, atorvastatin 20 mg daily, rosuvastatin 10 mg daily, pravastatin 40 mg daily and simvastatin 40 mg daily.

When do we use the new cholesterol-lowering medications like PCSK-9 inhibitors?

PCSK-9 inhibitors are a new group of cholesterol-lowering medications. They are very effective which can lower your LDL up to 77%, but they are very expensive.

Currently, we have two medications on the market, Repatha and Praluent. Only Repatha is licensed to treat homozygous familial hypercholesterolemia. Otherwise, both medications have the same indications.

FDA approved indications for anti-PCSK9 monoclonal antibodies in addition to diet and maximally tolerated statin therapy for additional LDL-C lowering.

	Clinical ASCVD*	Heterozygous FH	Homozygous FH
evolocumab (Repatha)	+	+	+
alirocumab (Praluent)	+	+	-

*Clinical ASCVD includes acute coronary syndromes, history of myocardial infarction, stable or unstable angina, coronary or other arterial revascularization, stroke, transient ischemic attack, or peripheral arterial disease presumed to be of atherosclerotic origin. See more at:

http://www.acc.org/latest-in-cardiology/articles/2016/05/18/14/34/current-indications-cost-and-clinical-use-of-anti-pcsk9-monoclonal-antibodies#sthash.4WNjtIfc.dpuf

Chapter 19: Diabetes and gastroparesis

My doctor said I have diabetic gastroparesis. What is it?

The stomach does a lot of work after we eat something. The stomach muscles aided by acid grind food into tiny, tiny pieces. The stomach muscle grinding is initiated by pacer and spread controlled by an internal nervous system. Usually, when eating a balanced meal, our stomachs will empty 60% of the food in 2 hours and empty completely in 4 hours. But if your stomach delays emptying and causes severe nausea, vomiting, early satiety, bloating and or upper abdominal pain, and then we say you might have gastroparesis

Does diabetes sometimes cause gastroparesis?

If your diabetes has not been controlled for a long time, you might develop diabetic neuropathy. If neuropathy is in your hands or feet, you will have numbness, tingling and or pain. If it is very severe, you might lose sensation completely. If neuropathy happens in your stomach, then your stomach can lose the ability to contract and move, and digest food properly.

How common is diabetic gastroparesis?

From a population study, gastroparesis is around 10% for those with type 1 diabetes over 10 years, for type 2 diabetes it is around 5%. The rate is much higher in people whose sugar has not been controlled.

How is gastroparesis diagnosed?

Usually for a concrete diagnosis, you need to see a gastroenterologist. You might need more tests to make sure you do not have other things going on in your gastrointestinal system. Your GI doctor will give you the detailed information.

Your gastroenterologists may ask you to take a test (scintigraphy) to determine the extent of gastroparesis (if any). This is a nuclear medicine test that shows how long it takes your stomach to empty its contents. You are given some special food to eat and the test measures how much of it remains in your stomach after four hours. The percentage remaining determines the level of gastroparesis. The three levels are:

- Mild gastroparesis: (10-15% of the food remained in stomach)
- Moderate gastroparesis: (15-35% of the food remained in stomach)
- Severe gastroparesis☹ >35% of the food remained in stomach)

Is there anything I need to know before my doctor gives me a diagnosis of gastroparesis?

First, before you go to have your stomach emptying test, you need to get your sugar under control. Since high sugar slows down your stomach, your sugar needs to be under 250 mg/dl on the day of testing.

Second, make sure you talk to your GI doctor about the medications you are taking which might cause gastroparesis.

Which medications can slow down gastric emptying?

In the diabetes world, metformin is the most common diabetes medication. Metformin can slow down gastric emptying and cause you to have nausea and vomiting. You might ask your doctor to see if you can stop taking it for a while.

The second most common medications that slow down gastric emptying are the GLP-1 agonists:

- Byetta
- Bydureon
- Trulicity
- Tanzeum.
- Combinations like Soliqua 100/33 or Xultophy.

More medications might come out. So, ask about those. For type 1 diabetes, Symlin (Amylin analogues) can also cause gastroparesis. All these drugs should be stopped.

Are there any medications other than diabetes medications that can delay gastric emptying?

Yes, there are many medications that can delay gastric emptying. This is why you need to talk to your doctor, including your GI doctor, to see if you can quit taking some of these medications.

Commonly used medications which can delay gastric emptying are:

- Blood pressure medications like alpha-2 adrenergic agonist like clonidine; calcium channel blockers like amlodipine, Cardene, nifedipine, cardizem.
- Tricyclic antidepressants- luckily these days, we do not use so often, like amitriptyline.
- Some medications, ironically, are used for abdominal pain, like hyoscyamine (Levbid), dicyclomine, Librax, and so on.

Are there any other medical conditions that can mimic gastroparesis?

Some other conditions might mimic gastroparesis. Such as,

- Some psychiatric diseases like depression, anxiety, anorexia nervosa, anorexia bulimia, psychogenic vomiting. Your doctor may have trouble differentiating them. You need to talk to your doctor about everything.
- Functional dyspepsia, which also has early satiety, postprandial fullness, and epigastric pain or burning. This condition can also have slow gastric emptying. Your GI doctor will figure it out for you.
- Cyclic vomiting syndrome. This is another difficult condition to treat and to differentiate. Patients suffering from this condition are characterized by episodes of intense nausea and vomiting lasting hours to days. These are separated by symptom-free periods of variable lengths.

Is there anything can I do to mitigate the symptoms?

Yes, you can do a lot. Here are some of my recommendations:

1. Focus on controlling your diabetes. Check your sugar and take your medicines as prescribed.
2. Do not drink any ice-cold water. The right temperature is important for your stomach to work. Many people are surprised that their stomach works much better after they begin to drink warm water. Think about it. If your stomach has been frozen, how can it move and perform its job of grinding?
3. Cook your food longer. Get a slow cooker. The more thoroughly you cook your food, the less your stomach needs to work. Even if you have severe gastroparesis, your stomach usually does not have trouble handling liquid.
4. Do not eat raw vegetables.
5. Invest in a good high-powered blender like Ninja. Let the machine do more work, and let your stomach do less work.
6. Ask your doctor to review all your medications to see if any of them can worsen your gastroparesis. For the medications which can cause or worsen gastroparesis, please see above.
7. Never ever eat pizza, chicken nuggets, or other high fat foods, especially high animal fat foods like red meat.
8. Do not drink sodas, lemon juice, or orange juice.
9. Do not eat high acidic foods like oranges, or food that is too spicy.
10. Do not eat too much at one meal. Never go to a buffet.
11. Try not to drink alcohol.
12. Certainly, no smoking. Smoking will slow down your stomach emptying. Some patients gain weight after they stop smoking. Stopping smoking is part of the reason they eat more.
13. Jogging and walking actually increase gastric motility. Always take a walk after a meal, but walk slowly.

Do I need to take extra vitamins for gastroparesis?

Yes, I recommend you to take sublingual vitamin B12, vitamin B6 and alpha lipoic acid. These vitamins can also help your diabetic neuropathy.

You need to prevent fat-soluble vitamin deficiency, especially vitamin D. Other lipid soluble vitamins are A, E and K. If possible, please take supplements for these. You might also develop thiamine and folate deficiency. Therefore, it is important to keep supplementing your diet with these vitamins.

My doctor put me on a medication called metoclopramide. When I read the side effects, they are very severe. Should I continue taking it?

This is the first-line of treatment for gastroparesis. It is a dopamine 2 receptor antagonist, a 5-HT 4 agonist, and a weak 5-HT3 receptor antagonist. It improves gastric emptying by enhancing gastric annular contractions and decreases postprandial gastric fundal relaxation. It is true that after long-term use this medication can have serious side effects. These side effects may include anxiety, restlessness, depression, hyperprolactinemia, QT interval prolongation and a condition called dyskinesia. Dyskinesia is characterized by involuntary movements of the tongue, lips, face, trunk and extremities.

You indeed must talk to your doctor if you need to take this medication on a long-term basis.

Domperidone was recommended to me, but it is not FDA approved in the US. Where can I buy it?

Domperidone is still not FDA approved since it can cause sudden death. It is recommended that you have an EKG before and during the treatment. You need to stop if your corrected QT interval is >470 ms if you are a man and if >450 ms if you are a woman. Domperidone has many drug interactions. It is legal in Canada, and many of my patients buy it from a

Canadian online pharmacy. You need to talk to your doctor before you use it.

How can macrolide antibiotics help relieve gastroparesis?

Macrolide antibiotics, like erythromycin or azithromycin induces high-amplitude gastric propulsive contractions that increase gastric emptying.

Can I take macrolide antibiotics long term?

No, you should not. You should not take these longer than four weeks at a time.

What are the risks of using macrolide antibiotics?

Long-term antibiotic use can induce antibiotic resistant strains. It might also cause gastrointestinal toxicity, hearing damage, or sudden death due to QT prolongation.

Why is cisapride not readily available in US?

Cisapride is a 5HT4 agonist which stimulates gastral and duodenal motility and accelerates gastric emptying of solids and liquids. Cisapride is better tolerated than metoclopramide, but its use has been associated with sudden death.

Why does my sugar vary widely from very low to very high?

Gastroparesis can make your diabetes control a nightmare, especially for someone with type 1 diabetes. Food that stays in the stomach is not digested, and their sugar might drop if their insulin is not adjusted properly.

Gastroparesis can also cause diabetic ketoacidosis that makes your nausea and vomiting worse. I have seen this happen in patients with type 1 diabetes when their sugar was not high and no insulin was given, or because they were not eating and no insulin was given, or not enough insulin was given. Because of nausea and vomiting, they are not drinking fluid and develop severe dehydration. The patient then develops diabetic ketoacidosis. The nausea and vomiting itself can also cause or worsen diabetic ketoacidosis.

Food that stays in the stomach too long might spoil and cause bacteria to grow and cause food poisoning. This can make the nausea and vomiting even worse.

Undigested food can harden and form a lump or a ball that is called a bezoar. This can cause obstructions which cause worsening nausea and vomiting.

Dehydration causes an electrolyte imbalance and may cause insulin resistance. Then, your sugar might go sky high.

What can we do about my unstable sugar?

If you have type 1 diabetes, you certainly are using insulin. Do not use any Amylin product. Any long-acting insulin is recommended. For fast-acting insulin, I recommend that you use regular insulin instead of analogs like Humalog, Novolog or Apidra. Regular insulin might match your prolonged food retention in the stomach.

Any time before you eat, check your sugar, and give a bolus properly.

If you have type 2 diabetes, stopping all oral medication is recommended. No oral medication is good for you. I recommended you start insulin also. Here are the reasons: metformin might cause worsening of your gastroparesis. SGLT2 antagonists cause dehydration which might lead to DKA. Sulphonylurea might cause severe hypoglycemia.

Check your sugar every time before you eat or when you feel your sugar is too high or too low.

Ideally, to stabilize your sugar you need an insulin pump and a CGM. We can use the special features of your pump to stabilize your sugar, and we can use CGM to monitor your sugar more closely.

Chapter 20: Diabetic foot care

Why should I check my feet every day?

Most diabetics have peripheral diabetic neuropathy and you can have a problem even before you realize it. Before it is too late, you need to check your feet every day. It is an important part of diabetes self-care.

I cannot see the bottom of my feet. What can I do?

Before going to bed or after a shower ask your loved one to check for you, or you can use a mirror. This does not take too long.

What daily foot care should I do?

You need to wash your feet with mild soap and warm water. Soaking your feet is not recommended since it might increase your chance of infection. It is very important to test the water temperature. It should be warm, not hot. Then dry your feet thoroughly including between your toes.

Why are my feet very dry and cracked?

This is because you have diabetic neuropathy, which causes the sweat glands not to work properly.

What brand is the best cream or moisturizer for diabetic dry feet?

Most patients who use Eucerin or Gold Bond Ultimate are satisfied. I have patients who use O'Keeffe's foot cream and have positive reviews.

What should I do if I find a small cut or scratches on my foot?

Again, if it is small, and if there is no sign of infection like severe redness, swelling or oozing secretion or pus, then you can wash it with clean warm water and a very gentle soap. Do this for the whole foot and dry it well. Look carefully any debris in the cut. If you see some debris, use a tweezers sterilized with alcohol to remove it. Apply a very thin layer of antibiotic cream like Neosporin, Polysporin or Bactroban. Then cover it with a bandage.

What should I do if I have a deep cut?

If you have any deep cut or any small cut on your foot, and you do not feel like you should take care of it yourself, go see your doctor or podiatrist.

When should I get a tetanus shot?

If you have a deep cut and your last tetanus shot was 5 years ago, you should talk to your doctor and get one.

What is the most important thing to do to prevent future cuts?

Examine the cut and think about it. Try to figure out why you got the cut in the first place. You need to have a pair of good shoes and good socks. You might be qualified to get a pair of diabetic shoes which can be fitted for you. Talk to your doctor and see a podiatrist.

When should I see a doctor for a cut?

You should see a doctor whenever you feel you need to see a doctor. Please trust your gut and see one. You should see a doctor when you have a deep cut, especially with redness, swelling, pain or a wound oozing with pus. You should see a doctor for any wound you managed yourself and then it did not get better.

I have a blister on my foot. What should I do?

If the blister is small, look carefully at your shoes to see if anything there caused it, and do not wear that shoe again. You might need to see a podiatrist to make sure your shoes and socks are a good fit for you. If the blister is small, you do not need to drain it. It will be absorbed in a few days as long as the cause is removed.

However, if the blister is big, and if there is a good chance it will break on its own, I recommend you drain the blister.

Here's how:

1. Wash your hands and the blister with soap and warm water. Swab the blister with iodine if you have it. It is okay if you do not have it. You can use 70% alcohol.
2. Find a clean, sharp unused needle.
3. Use the needle to puncture the blister. Aim for several spots near the blister's edge. Let the fluid drain, but leave the overlying skin in place.
4. Apply an ointment (Vaseline, Plastibase, Bactroban, Neosporin, or others) to the blister and cover it with a nonstick gauze bandage. If a rash appears, stop using the ointment.
5. Change the dressing every day. Apply more ointment and a bandage.

I have calluses. What should I do?

A callus is not something you should take care of yourself, since if not properly taken care of, it might lead to infection and a foot ulcer. Go to see a podiatrist and let a professional take care of it. The podiatrist will help you to get a pair of therapeutic diabetic shoes and good support inserts. These will prevent future calluses.

I just found an ulcer on my foot. What should I do?

If you had followed my instructions for foot care, you might not have one today. Hopefully, this is your wake-up call to check your sugar and eat right to get your sugar in better control.

First, you need to keep it clean and see a podiatrist for wound care as soon as you can. Based on the severity, you might need antibiotics, wound cleaning, debridement, or off-loading. There is no way you can take care of an ulcer yourself. You need to see a doctor. This is really important if you have fever or oozing pus. The ulcer might cause a blood infection or a bone infection, and it needs to be taken care of by a doctor as soon as you can.

No matter what I do, I have freezing cold feet. Is there anything you can suggest?

Cold feet can be very annoying and cold feet can decrease your quality of life. Your feet can feel cold even when the rest of your body is very hot. I call it "cold feet syndrome." A small fraction of patients have vascular problems (circulation problems), but most people have diabetic neuropathy.

First, you can try Capsaicin cream. You can buy it from drugstores like CVS or Walgreens. If this is not effective, your doctor might try Gabapentin or Lyrica. Wearing warm socks always helps, but usually this cannot solve the problem.

Here is one thing you should never do. Do not stick your feet in hot water that might burn your feet and cause infection. It is okay to warm your feet with warm water bottles and heating pads with appropriate temperature.

If you have a circulation problem with the big vessels in your feet, we call this peripheral vascular disease. We can test for this and confirm it. If you have small vessel disease we cannot even test for it.

If the above measures are not effective, your doctor should test you for peripheral vascular disease and treat it accordingly, especially if you have pain and it becomes worse after walking.

I have found that I have a black toe. What should I do?

Hopefully, you knew this before. Diabetic vascular problems, such as peripheral vascular disease, can cause an ulcer or gangrene. Sometimes when this happens, amputation is the only solution. Therefore, take care of yourself. Check your sugar and take your medications as prescribed. Do not wait until it is too late.

I have diabetic neuropathy and I have burning pain in my feet. It is so bad that I cannot sleep. What should I do?

Diabetic neuropathy can be very challenging to treat and can significantly reduce your quality of life. Therefore, I always recommend to my patients that they should care for their diabetes seriously.

Here are some things you can do to help your neuropathy:

1. Your doctor should do a careful foot exam to make sure there are no other foot complications. Make sure there are no other conditions besides diabetes that would worsen your diabetic neuropathy. Many diabetes patients also have heart failure, obesity and vein insufficiency. These can cause severe bilateral low extremity swelling. The swelling can compromise the small vessel circulation and worsen the neuropathy. The swelling needs to be treated. Otherwise, the other measures might not be effective.
2. I would try some over the counter vitamins, such as B12, B6 and lipoic acid.
3. If this is still not working, I would try a prescription vitamin like Metanx which contains an active form of folic acid and vitamins B6 and B12.
4. If this is still not effective, I would try Gabapentin or Lyrica.
5. Some patients have found SSRI or SNRI to be helpful.
6. I have patients who have used all of above but still cannot get relief.
7. Lidocaine spray can be tried. Other creams like Capsaicin might also be used as an adjunctive treatment.

Again, taking care of your diabetes is the best way to avoid all these troubles.

Chapter 21: Diabetes and sexual dysfunction

How common is the problem of sexual dysfunction in men with diabetes?

It is well known that men with diabetes have a very high risk for erectile dysfunction. It is estimated that about 35% to 75% of these men will experience at least some degree of erectile dysfunction (ED) during their lifetime.

Men with diabetes tend to develop erectile dysfunction 10 to 15 years earlier than men without diabetes. As men with diabetes age, erectile dysfunction becomes even more common. The likelihood of having difficulty with an erection occurs in approximately 50% to 60% of men with diabetes for men over 50. Above age 70, there is about a 95% likelihood of having some difficulty with erectile dysfunction.

Why do men with diabetes have erectile dysfunction?

Successful erections need the nerves and blood vessels to work together. If the nerves or blood vessels have problems, it will lead to erectile dysfunction. As we know, long-term diabetes can cause diabetic neuropathy and cardiovascular disease.

I am over 60, why should I care about sex?

It is normal to have slightly reduced libido as you age, but even men in their 90s can still have normal sexual function. Sexual dysfunction can affect your mood, motivation, self-esteem and relationships profoundly. As we discussed above, erectile dysfunction can be a sign of cardiovascular disease. You might also need to alert your doctor and be tested for this.

I am embarrassed. How should I raise this issue with my doctor?

Your doctor should ask this question, but more often, he or she does not. Your doctor is being pressed by Medicare and the insurance companies to treat more patients. The insurance companies are less concerned about patient wellbeing than your doctor. Your doctor's time is focused on your blood pressure, cholesterol, blood sugar, and A1c.

You need to be your own advocate and raise this issue to your doctor if he or she does not ask you about it.

As we discussed above, you are not alone. If you are above 50 and have had diabetes for at least 10 years, your chance of having ED is over 50%. So, just be direct with your doctor and tell him or her that you have ED.

What can I do to prevent ED?

Here are a few things you can do:

1. Try your best to work with your doctor to get your diabetes under control. There is a direct correlation between the A1c and ED.
2. Stop smoking if you are a smoker.
3. Make diet, exercise and life-style changes to make sure your weight is under control.
4. Take your statins as prescribed.

Should I stop drinking?

Yes, you should. Alcohol can cause ED or make ED worse.

What should I do if I have ED?

Here are seven recommendations:

1. Raise this issue with your doctor, as we discussed. This might indicate you have a more serious condition like cardiovascular

disease. Your doctor might refer you to a cardiologist to have a test.
2. Stop smoking. If you smoke, it's never too late to quit.
3. Talk to your partner. Help your partner understand this can be caused by diabetes or cardiovascular disease. Let your partner know you are struggling with it. Tell your partner this is not because you have less love, or that your sexual needs are being met from somewhere else. Your partner's understanding and support plays a very important part in making sure you can succeed.
4. Ask your doctor to review your medications. There is a long list of medications that can cause or worsen ED. Some medications may be able to be discontinued or changed.
5. Get the gear to get yourself in shape.
6. Try your best to follow a good diabetic regimen to get it under control.
7. You might ask to try medications like Viagra, Levitra, Cialis, Stendra, etc.

Is there anything else I can do if my insurance does not pay for Viagra, Levitra, Stendra, or Cialis?

It is sad now how your insurance dictates your treatment. The good news is Viagra is now generic. It is available for pulmonary hypertension. You can ask your doctor for it. It is not available in all pharmacies.

Can I buy ED drugs online?

The standard answer is NO. Apparently you are running a risk of not getting the pure medication, not the right dose, contamination and all sorts of other issues. You may not know what you are truly taking.

Again, nowadays, due to the insurance, patients are being squeezed and pushed. I understand your pain. You have to take your own risks. I have anecdotal evidence for both sides of the issue.

Are there any herbs I can try?

There is no standard trial to confirm any herbs work for this purpose. The common supplements people are trying are:

1. Ginkgo biloba is an herb from a Chinese tree. Your risk for bleeding may increase, especially if you are on blood thinning medications. So do not start this on your own. You need to talk to your doctor before you start.
2. Ginseng is very popular in Asia, especially, in China.
3. Rhodiola Rosea.
4. L-arginine is an amino acid which is the substrate to make nitric oxide. This is the gas which was found to relax penis blood vessels. The effectiveness and side effects have not been well-defined.

Acupuncture is known to stimulate the nerves which are important to regulate penis blood supply.

What do I need to know before I try prescription medications like Viagra, Levitra, Stendra, and Cialis?

If you have cardiovascular disease and you are taking nitrates, you should not take them. It might cause very severe low blood pressure which could be life threatening. The same thing is true if you have taken an ED medication in the past 24 hour. If you have chest pain, make sure you tell the physician who is treating you.

Other side effects include, but are not limited to, headaches, flushing, nasal congestion, indigestion and vision impairment.

Is there anything I can do about my performance anxiety?

Sometimes, anxiety is a big issue. Actually, the best way to overcome anxiety is to talk it through with your sexual partner and get her understanding. This can ease your anxiety. Certainly, if a good sex therapist is available in your area, you can try that.

Should I have my doctor check my testosterone?

Testosterone certainly plays a very important role in sexual function. It is extremely important for libido. It also has a permissive role for erection.

The decrease in testosterone in diabetes is mostly due to secondary causes. You may have depression, chronic pain, obstructive sleep apnea, stress, or poor sleep. The medications used to treat these and other conditions might reduce your testosterone. Also, testosterone is converted to estrogen in fat cells by an enzyme called aromatase.

It is very reasonable to have your doctor check your testosterone.

When should I check my testosterone?

You should have your doctor check your testosterone early in the morning. Testosterone secretion has a diurnal pattern. It is highest early in the morning.

My testosterone was at a low level. Should I get it treated?

You should be evaluated by an endocrinologist. Please do not go to a testosterone clinic. I personally found at least five pituitary tumors which were being wrongly treated with injectable testosterone. This is beyond the discussion of this book.

Chapter 22: Living with someone who has diabetes

What are the challenges in families with someone who has diabetes?

Diabetes is a difficult disease since it is with you all the time. It is not an acute disease, but if you do not take care of it, it can become acute and an emergency at any time. Sometimes, you seem to be doing all the right things, but things still can go wrong. You have an emergency, and you might think it just belongs to you. No, it affects everyone surrounding you, especially those who love you. Diabetes can cause much stress on you and your loved ones. It takes time for you and your loved ones to adapt, to learn and to improve.

How can I help my spouse to understand the disease?

If the diagnosis comes after your marriage, your spouse might be shocked, scared and stressed like you. Your spouse can have the same feelings as yours, such as denial, shame, guilt, and depression. The first important thing is to accept it. Only after you accept it, then you can take steps to deal with it. Let your spouse know this is no one's fault, and you are not alone. In 2014, there were 29 million Americans who had diabetes, and 86 million who had prediabetes.

Another good thing is for both of you to go to your diabetes educator together and read this book together. It might even be better if you get another copy of this book for your spouse. This may help your spouse understand your problems even more.

My spouse is always nagging me about my diabetes. What can I do?

You are lucky that you have someone who cares enough to nag you. Sometimes, if you live alone, it can be dangerous for diabetes. You need to understand that your spouse might still be scared about this disease. He or she is worrying about you and worrying about your future. If your diabetes has not been controlled for a long time, the risk for blindness, amputations, kidney failure, heart attacks and strokes will increase significantly.

You need to sit down and talk to your spouse when things are calm. You need to assure him or her that you are taking diabetes seriously. You need to make an agreement with your spouse about what you want your spouse to help you with. Also, let him or her know what you do not want help with. Let your spouse know that the unwanted help is creating resentment, and it is not helping your diabetes at all.

When should I listen to my spouse?

One feature of diabetes is that your sugar might be unstable. You might change your mood. Let your spouse know your mental status might change, and you might have behavior changes. You might not know it at all. It can really save your life if you listen to your spouse to check your sugar in moments like these. This is my general recommendation: if your spouse thinks you need to check your sugar, you are better off if you check it.

My spouse is like the "diabetes police," I feel like a criminal who is under surveillance 24 hours a day. I hate this. What can I do?

You should be appreciative that you have someone to police you. Like anywhere else, if you do not have police, the situation will be chaotic and you do not want to live there. I have many patients that do not have any police and they are living in fear. As I said, diabetes can be scary if you never know if your sugar might be too high or too low. I bet you heard before of something called "DIB." This stands for **D**ied **I**n **B**ed. People do not know what is happening to them, and now they are dead.

Again, what you can do on a good day is to sit down with your spouse and talk about it. You can make an agreement about what you need to be policed on and what you do not need to be policed on. This is the best you can do, since you have to understand that your spouse is worried and scared also.

I lost my libido. What should I do?

This is very common. This is especially true if your diabetes has not been well-controlled. Diabetes can cause lots of stress and fatigue. You can become overwhelmed by all of this and experience decreased libido. For females, poorly controlled diabetes can cause UTI or vaginal yeast infections. These conditions certainly may take away female libido.

Therefore, taking care of your diabetes is very important.

Again, sit down and talk to your spouse. Let your spouse know this might be caused by diabetes. It is not due to your spouse's lack of attraction or love. Talk to your doctor about this. Your doctor might be able to pinpoint the cause and help you.

I still have libido, but I have ED. What can I do?

As we discussed it is very common to have ED in diabetes. Do not keep this to yourself, let both of you work together. You might have other ways to enjoy your sex life. The understanding of your spouse is crucial to ease your anxiety, guilt and anger. Therefore, talk about it and look at the options you have.

If you read this, and you do not have any problem with ED, good for you. You need to take care of your diabetes, and you can reduce your risk of developing ED. Again, bring your spouse with you and talk to your doctor during your visits.

Since my diagnosis of diabetes, my spouse prepares salads for every meal. I feel like a rabbit. I hate the food. What can I do?

As you know eating is crucial to control diabetes. Salads are a very important part of your diabetes diet. You need to get used to it.

You might also buy some diabetes cookbooks. You can prepare some food yourself or with your spouse. Learn together. There are many different dishes which are good for your diabetes and taste good. The point is to explore. Do not make a conclusion before you even start. The search for your new food can be fun and exciting. Bring your spouse to the diabetic education meetings and to your diabetes doctor's visits. Learning together is very important.

My spouse now prepares two sets of meals, one for me, which is very bland, and one for everyone else, which is all the food I like. I cannot resist eating their food. What can I do?

It is very lucky that you have someone who cares enough to prepare a special meal for you. You need to give the other family members and your spouse time to adapt to the diet you need to be on. While you are appreciating your spouse's effort, this does not mean you cannot discuss it. Your diet is healthier. One day, ideally, the whole family may eat the same.

However, the truth is that you can eat everything and anything you want to eat. The issue is the amount you eat and portion control. You are allowed to taste the food which is prepared for the rest of your family, but you should not eat too much of it.

I am feeling that I am dragging my spouse and whole family down. I am depressed. What should I do?

In research studies, patients with diabetes are reported to be 1.4 to 3 times more likely to suffer with depression than others without diabetes. Depression might lead a patient to develop diabetes. On the other hand, diabetes can lead to depression. This is a serious issue. I think you need to discuss this with your spouse and seek professional help.

Depression in diabetes is persistent and often recurrent. In longitudinal and follow-up studies the rates of depression persistence or recurrence have been reported to range widely, between 11.6% and 92%. These results depend on sample sizes, depression diagnosis criteria and depression classification (major depression or elevated depressive symptoms).

Again, diabetes can have a huge psychological burden on you and your spouse. Get as much help as you can from your parents, siblings and children, but try your best not to drag them down. Again, recognize this problem and seek help as soon as possible.

Chapter 23: Questions about diabetes emergencies

How to prevent low sugar and how to treat low sugar have been discussed in other chapters in this book. Here we are going to focus on two other diabetic emergencies—diabetes ketoacidosis (DKA) and hyperosmolar hyperglycemic state (HHS).

What is diabetic ketoacidosis?

Our body needs a certain acid level, hydration and electrolytes to work properly. Our body is amazing. It can keep all of these in a balanced status under normal conditions.

Normally, our body breaks down sugar as a source of energy. In this process, insulin is required. As you now know in type 1 diabetes, insulin is deficient. If our body does not have enough insulin, then our body cannot use sugar and our body will break down fat for our energy. The problem is that it breaks down too much and exceeds our body's ability to use them. The product of fat breakdown is ketones which is acid. Too much ketone buildup in the body is toxic. They make your body very acidic which makes your body not work properly. They (the ketones) and increased sugar also drag out lots water from your body which make your body very dehydrated.

Diabetic ketoacidosis is a serious problem. It can happen to people with either type 1 or type 2 diabetes, but it is more likely to affect people with type 1.

What is the mortality rate for DKA?

DKA is a serious complication of diabetes associated with significant mortality and high healthcare costs. The overall DKA mortality in the US is less than 1%, but a rate higher than 5% is reported in the elderly and in patients with concomitant, life-threatening illnesses.

What other damage might DKA do to your body?

DKA is an emergency. Many long-term effects have not been well-studied, but evidence has shown that repeated DKAs certainly damage a patient's brain and also increase long-term MACE (major adverse cardiac events).

Mortality in patients with HHS is reported between 5% and 16%, which is about 10 times higher than the mortality in patients with DKA.

What causes diabetic ketoacidosis?

People can get diabetic ketoacidosis for a few reasons:
1. **It is not known that you have diabetes.** Quite a high percentage of patients are diagnosed with type 1 diabetes because they are presented as DKA. A study from Colorado data between 1998 and 2012 determined diabetic ketoacidosis was present in 1,339 of 3,439 youth (38.9%) at type 1 diabetes diagnosis. Youth with DKA had a median age of 9.4 years (interquartile range, 5.6-12.6 years), 53.8% were male, and 75.7% were white.
2. **Patients forget to take insulin.** I also have patients who cannot pay for insulin, or they just do not take it when they should.
3. **Patients do not check their sugar.** If sugar is not checked regularly, and patients do not give insulin or do not give enough insulin.
4. **Insulin pump failure.** This also includes user errors such as not changing an infusion set or kinked tubing, or scar formation at the insertion site and gastrointestinal infection.
5. **Major health problem.** The patient might have a major illness or health problem, such as a heart attack or infection.
6. Taking certain medicines or illegal drugs.
7. **Patients do not take their insulin as directed.**
8. **Taking an SGLT2 medication.** Now, we have a new type 2 diabetes medication called SGLT2 inhibitors (see other section for

details); The FDA warns that this category of medication might cause type 2 diabetes to have normal sugar DKA.

What are the symptoms of diabetic ketoacidosis?

The symptoms can include but are not limited to the following, and the patient can have some or all of them. Symptoms can also start gradually and get worse Including:

1. Feeling very thirsty and drinking a lot of water.
2. Urinating a lot, including at night.
3. Nausea or vomiting is very common.
4. Belly pain.
5. Feeling tired or having trouble thinking clearly.
6. Having breath that smells sweet or fruity.
7. If severe enough and not treated, patients can have confusion and loss of consciousness and even death.

Should I see a doctor?

This is a life-threatening emergency. You need to go to the ER.

Is there anything I can do to prevent diabetic ketoacidosis?

Yes. Here are six recommendations for preventing DKA.

1. Take care of your diabetes. Eat and exercise right and take your insulin as prescribed.
2. Monitor your blood sugar levels. This is the key to keeping you out of trouble. You also need to have a plan to react to your high and low readings. If you do not have a plan, talk to your doctor.
3. Adjust your insulin dosage as needed. Again, it is very good for you to check your sugar, but is just as important that you need to know what

to do about these numbers. Please see my other sections, about how to respond to high sugar.

4. Check your ketone level. When you are ill or under stress, test your urine for excess ketones with an over-the-counter urine ketone test kit. If your ketone level is moderate or high, especially if you have other symptoms of DKA (see above), you definitely need to go to the ER.

5. If you have type 2 diabetes, and if you are taking one of the new SGLT2 inhibitor medications, you need to stop your medication and keep yourself well-hydrated. When you go to the ER, you need to let your treating physician know what you are taking.

6. Know what medication you have to take and what medication you can stop temporarily. When your doctor starts you on a new medication, you need to know when you need to stop and when you should not stop taking it.

How is diabetic ketoacidosis treated?

You need to go to the hospital to be treated.

- **Replenish fluids and correct electrolytes.** In DKA, patients lose a lot of fluid and also have electrolyte disturbances.
- **Take Insulin.** When the body has enough insulin, your body will start to use sugar as fuel and suppress your body from producing more ketones. Gradually your excess ketones will be metabolized and the acidic condition will be corrected.

What is a hyperosmolar hyperglycemic state (HHS)?

A hyperosmolar hyperglycemic state is another life-threatening diabetic emergency. This mostly occurs in type 2 diabetes patients. Our bodies are designed to have everything balanced and maintained in a very narrow normal range.

If the sugar gets too high, the sugar will pull water out of the cells and out of the body. This can cause the body's metabolism to be severely deranged.

What are the symptoms of a hyperosmolar hyperglycemic state?

A hyperosmolar hyperglycemic state can cause severe fatigue, disorientation, passing out (losing consciousness) and coma. But before that happens, people usually have symptoms for a few days that include:

- Urinating much more than usual
- Being very thirsty, and drinking much more than usual
- Losing weight
- Having dark yellow or brown urine

What are the factors which can cause a hyperosmolar hyperglycemic state?

HHS can be caused by several factors:

- Getting an infection or severe fever illness, especially a GI tract illness. This will usually cause nausea, vomiting and diarrhea.
- Having a heart attack or stroke.
- Stopping diabetes medicines or not taking the diabetes medicines as directed.
- Taking other medicines that affect sugar levels like high dose steroids.
- Becoming dehydrated. This is when the body loses too much water.

Is there a test for a hyperosmolar hyperglycemic state?

Yes.

Regularly check your sugar. If your sugar is consistently higher than 500, and you are not able to get it down, you need to go to hospital.

The hospital will do the tests to determine if you are in a hyperosmolar hyperglycemic state.

What can I do to prevent a hyperosmolar hyperglycemic state?

1. Take care of your diabetes. Eat and exercise right and take your insulin or your oral medications as prescribed.
2. Monitor your blood sugar levels. This is the key to keeping you out of trouble. You also need to have a plan to react to your readings. If you do not have a plan, talk to your doctor. It is also very important to know under what circumstances you need to stop taking certain medications.
3. Adjust your insulin dosage as needed. If you are taking insulin, it is important to know what you can do to get your sugar down under certain circumstances. Again, it is very good for you to check your sugar, but it is as important that you know what you should do about these numbers. Please see my other section, about how to respond to high sugar.
4. Check your ketone levels. A hyperosmolar hyperglycemic state usually occurs in adults with type 2 diabetes, but you need to check your ketones, too. When you are ill or under stress, test your urine for excess ketones with an over-the-counter urine ketones test kit. If your ketone level is moderate or high, especially if you have other symptoms of HHS (see above), you definitely need to go to the ER.
5. When you have high sugar and shortness of breath, chest pain and you feel very sick, you certainly need to go to the ER
6. Know what medication you have to take and what medication you can stop temporarily. When your doctor starts you on a new medication, you need to know when you need to stop taking it, and when you should not stop taking it.
7. Always keep yourself well hydrated.
8. If you have a GI tract disease or gastroparesis, and if you are not able to keep water and food down, you need to go to see your

doctor as soon as possible. You are usually given IV fluids which can prevent you from getting into full-blown hyperosmolar hyperglycemic state.

How is a hyperosmolar hyperglycemic state treated?

Patients with a hyperosmolar hyperglycemic state are treated in the hospital. These patients have severe dehydration and electrolyte disturbances.

- Fluids and electrolytes – In a hyperosmolar hyperglycemic state, the body loses a lot of fluids.
- Insulin is also given intravenously to get the sugar down slowly.
- The doctor will also treat any infection or illness causing the hyperosmolar hyperglycemic state.

Final Words

What are your final words on diabetes?

You actually have a big part to play in taking care of your diabetes. It is not all up to your doctor. You have the biggest part to play in taking care of your diabetes. This can be very challenging. However, there are many things you can do to make diabetes self-care work for you.

The ADA (American Diabetes Association) recommends the following seven self-care guidelines. If you follow these guidelines, you will greatly improve your overall diabetes care results.

1. **Healthy eating.** This is absolutely the most important of the seven. If your eating is not fixed, your diabetes can never be controlled no matter what medications you use. As I discussed, I recommend a low-meat, low-carb, high-fiber diet.
2. **Being active.** Being active is not just exercising. What I mean is that if you can stand, do not sit. If you can move around, do not stand still. Keep moving and do activities that require moving like cleaning, gardening, cooking, shopping, etc.
3. **Monitoring.** Check your sugar as recommended. Check your ketones as needed. Check your blood pressure as required. Also, make sure your doctor monitors your A1c, cholesterol, urine protein, etc.
4. **Taking medications.** Take the medications you are supposed to take, and know when and why you need to take them. If you are not taking the medications you are supposed to take, this can mislead your treating doctor. This might cause your doctor to make the wrong assumptions and hurt you eventually. I have a patient who is supposed to take long-acting insulin every day, but he did not follow the regimen due to financial difficulties. He took his insulin every other day. His sugar was not controlled, and then

his doctor increased his insulin all the way to over 300 units daily. His sugar was up and down. If, for some reason, you cannot take your medication as you are supposed to, you need to let your treating doctor know, and the regimen or medication needs to be changed. Your doctor can help you make the right changes.

5. **Risk reduction.** If you are a smoker, strive to quit. Make sure you have a yearly dilated eye exam. Check your own feet every day. Have regular podiatrist visits. Have all the vaccines you are supposed to have, like a yearly flu vaccine. Other vaccines like hepatitis B, pneumonia and shingles are also recommended for patients at different ages.

6. **Problem solving**. Life is complicated. Life is even more complicated with diabetes. Strive to learn problem-solving skills. Different problems pop up all the time. Try to learn about diabetes as much as possible, so you can manage it better. Then you will not have to be panic when difficult situations arise.

7. **Healthy coping.** Again, dealing with diabetes is very challenging, and it is normal to have different emotions. Make sure you do not to let depression, frustration or anxiety affect you management of diabetes.

Appendix: A list of all 400+ questions in this book

Chapter 1: Essentials you need to know after being newly diagnosed with diabetes 1

Diet and exercise questions 1
What can I eat? 1
How should I eat? 2
What can I do for exercise? 3
How much weight should I lose? 4
A1c questions 4
Diabetes patients are talking about A1c. What is it? 4
What is my target A1c? 5
Is the A1c goal different for those with CAD? 5
How often should I check my A1c? 5
Blood sugar monitoring questions 6
How often and when should I check my sugar? 6
Questions about glucometers 9
Which glucometer do you recommend? 9
Which glucometer is most accurate? 10
I would like to have a talking meter. Which meters can do that? 10
When should I change my glucometer? 11
How do I know if my meter is accurate or not? 11
I have financial difficulties. What can I do to lower my cost for strips? 11
I am checking my sugar 20 times a day. Do you have any recommendations for me? 12
Insulin pump and monitoring questions 13
I have an insulin pump. Do you have a meter which can send the sugar information to the pump directly? 13

Are there meters that can send my blood sugar to my phone, iPad or computer wirelessly? 13
Are there meters that can be plugged into a computer via USB directly? 13
When should I look into CGM (continuous glucose monitoring)?..........14
Which CGM is the best? 14
Blood sugar, cholesterol and weight targets 15
What sugar target should I shoot for? 15
What is my cholesterol target level? 16
What should my blood pressure target be? 16

Chapter 2: 10 questions to ask your insurance company about diabetes coverage 17

Does my insurance policy cover diabetes self-management education? 17
Does my insurance company sponsor any community programs for healthy lifestyle changes? 17
What kind of glucometer does it cover? 17
What diabetes medications are in the formulary? 18
What cholesterol medications does it cover? 18
Does my insurance cover ophthalmologist's (eye doctor) visits? 18
Does my insurance cover podiatrist's (foot doctor) visits? 18
Does my insurance cover weight loss? 18
Does my insurance cover continuous glucose monitoring (CGM)? 19
Does my insurance cover insulin pumps?...................................19

Chapter 3: 10 things to discuss with your family about diabetes 20

When should I share my diabetes diagnosis with my family and friends? 20
What should I let my family know about my diet? 20
What should I let my family know about my drinks?................20
What does my family need to know about exercise? 21

What does my family need to know about my new routine? 21

What does my family need to know about diabetes medications? 21

How do my family and I know if I have low blood sugar? 22

Should I teach my family members how to check my sugar? 22

How should I handle glucagon shots? 22

Do I need to tell my family about A1c and what my A1c target is? 23

Chapter 4: 10 questions to ask before starting a new medication 24

What is the necessity of starting a new medication? 24

Does it have a generic version? 24

How will it help my diabetes? 24

Does it have interactions with other medications I am taking? 25

What side effects do I need to watch for? 25

When should I stop or adjust the dose? 25

Should I take my medications before a meal, with a meal, or after a meal, or at bedtime? 25

Can I double my dose if my sugar is too high? 26

Can I continue my medication if I am going to have a CT scan or cardiac catheterization? 26

What should I do if I am going to have a procedure like a colonoscopy or surgery? 26

Chapter 5: The basics of diabetes 27

Questions about diabetes prevention 27

Can diabetes be prevented? 27

How can I prevent diabetes? 27

Does weight loss reduce my risk of developing diabetes from prediabetes? 27

Does lifestyle modification and metformin reduce my risk of developing diabetes? 27

Can rosiglitazone or pioglitazone be used for diabetes prevention? 28

Is acarbose effective for diabetes prevention? 28
Can Xenical/Alli prevent diabetes? 28
Can estrogen prevent diabetes? 28
Does vitamin D prevent diabetes? 28
Can cinnamon prevent diabetes? 29
Does stopping smoking prevent diabetes? 29
Can bariatric surgery prevent diabetes? 29
Can bariatric surgery cure type 2 diabetes? 29
Is it true the "Little Blue Pill" Viagra can prevent diabetes? 29
Does more or less sleep prevent diabetes? 29
Can CPAP (breathing machine) reduce diabetes? 30
Diabetes screening questions 30
Who should be screened for diabetes? 30
How do we screen for diabetes? 30
How do we do the OGTT? 31
Questions about the different types of diabetes 31
What is diabetes? 31
What is insulin resistance? 32
What is prediabetes? 32
What is type 1 diabetes? 32
What is type 2 diabetes? 32
What is type 3 diabetes? 33
What is type 1.5 diabetes? 33
What is LADA? 33
What is gestational diabetes? 34
Can children have type 2 diabetes? 34
Can adults have type 1 diabetes? 34
Are there any other types of diabetes? 34
What is steroid induced diabetes? 34

What is "brown diabetes"? 35
Questions about other causes of diabetes 35
Do night shifts cause diabetes? 35
Do sugary drinks really cause diabetes? 35
Do plastic products cause diabetes? 35
Questions about diagnosing diabetes 36
How do doctors tell if I have type 1 or type 2 diabetes? 36
What are the symptoms of diabetes? 36
Why does my doctor say I have diabetes, but I do not have any symptoms? 36
How is diabetes diagnosed? 36
Questions about the risk of diabetes 37
If my brother or sister has type 1 diabetes, what are the chances for me to have type 1 diabetes? 37
If my twin brother or sister has type 1 diabetes, what is the chance for me to have type 1 diabetes? 37
If a parent has type 1 diabetes, what is the risk for a child to develop type 1 diabetes? 37
Is race/ethnicity a risk factor for developing diabetes? 38
My sibling was diagnosed with type 2 diabetes. What is my chance to get it? 38
If my parent has type 2 diabetes and my sibling also develops diabetes, what is my risk? 38
If both my parents have type 2 diabetes and one of my siblings developed diabetes, what are my odds of developing diabetes? 39
My spouse developed type 2 diabetes. Is my risk increased? 39
Questions about doctors and doctor's visits 39
What are some questions I should ask my doctor about diabetes treatment? 39
What do I do if I don't like my current doctor? 40

Are there any doctors that specialize in diabetes care? 41

How do I choose a good diabetes doctor?...42

Chapter 6: Diabetic education 44

When should I get diabetic education? 44

What can I learn from diabetic education?...44

What do I need to do to prepare for one-on-one diabetes education? 44

Chapter 7: How is type 1 diabetes treated? 46

Questions about curing type 1 diabetes 46

Can we cure type 1 diabetes with a pancreas transplant?.........................46

Where can I get an islet transplant or a beta cell transplant? 46

How far away is the artificial pancreas?..47

Questions about medications, insulin pumps and monitoring................47

Are there oral medications for type 1 diabetes?..47

Are insulin pumps better than multiple daily injections?.........................48

Which insulin pump is the best?...48

How can I motivate my child to check his or her sugar? 49

Questions about high and low blood sugar levels.....................................50

Why does my sugar increase after exercising? 50

Why does my sugar decrease after exercising?...50

What symptoms or signs might indicate low sugar? 50

What should I do if I feel my sugar is low?..51

How should I treat low sugar?...51

What should I do if my sugar is low and I do not feel it? 51

What should I do if I cannot feel when my sugar is low? 52

My morning sugar is always high. What can I do? 53

When should I use the glucagon shot my doctor prescribed for me? 54

How should I use the glucagon shot?..54

When do I need to check urine sugar?...55

Questions about ketones, high sugar and diabetic ketoacidosis (DKA) . 55

When do I need to check urine ketones? 55

What do I need to do if my ketones are positive? 56

What should I do if I have nausea and vomiting and I am unable to keep anything down? 56

What should I do if my sugar goes above 500 after a steroid shot? 56

What should I do if my sugar goes over 500 and I am not taking steroids? 57

What are the common reasons for sugar to go over 500? 57

What should I do if for no reason my sugar goes over 500? 57

What should I do if my sugar is persistently higher than 250 and I do not feel well? 58

Chapter 8: How is type 2 diabetes treated? 59

What is metformin? 59

Why is metformin so popular? 59

Is it true that metformin might have a brain benefit? 60

What are the brand names for metformin? 60

I cannot take the big pill. What can I do? 60

I cannot tolerate the regular metformin. What options do I have? 60

I swear I saw a big pill in my stool? Has this happened with other people? 61

Does metformin cause vitamin B12 deficiency? 61

Does metformin cause renal failure? 62

Does metformin cause heart failure? 62

Does metformin cause lactic acidosis? 62

When should I temporarily stop metformin? 62

What is the best medication for type 2 diabetes? 63

Which oral medication is prone to cause hypoglycemia? 62

Why are sulfonylureas not so popular now? 63

Why did my doctor switch me from glyburide to glimepiride?............63
Should I stop taking sulfonylureas? 64
Do sulfonylureas cause more heart attacks? 64
What are DPP-4 inhibitors? 64
What are the DDP-4 inhibitors currently on the market?..........................65
Which DPP-4 inhibitor is the best? 65
What should I know before I begin to take a DPP-4 inhibitor?................66
I heard that DPP-4 inhibitors cause heart failure. Is it true? 66
When should I temporarily stop a DPP4-inhibitor? 67
What are GLP-1 agonists? 67
What are the currently GLP-1 agonists on the market?.............................67
Which GLP-1 agonist is the best?...68
How to adjust the dose of Victoza? 68
What should I know before I begin to take GLP-1 agonist?......................69
What should I do if I have too much nausea when I take a GLP-1 agonist?...70
What is an SGLT2 inhibitor? 71
Which SGLT2 inhibitors are currently on the market?..............................71
Which SGLT2 inhibitor is the best?..72
What should I know before I begin to take SGLT2 inhibitors? 72
What can I do to reduce the chances for UTIs or yeast infections?..........73
Does SGLT2 reduce cardiovascular risk in type 2 diabetes? 73
Lawyers have Ads on TV, should I stop the medication? 74
When should I temporarily stop an SGLT2 antagonist? 74
What is acarbose?..75
What are the adverse effects of acarbose? 75
How do I reduce the side effects of flatulence and diarrhea? 75
What should I do if I have lots of gas when I take acarbose? 75
When should I temporarily stop taking acarbose? 75

I have type 2 diabetes, why does my doctor prescribe insulin for me? .. 76
What is the best insulin that I should take for type 2 diabetes? 76
What kind of insulin can I use for type 2 diabetes? 76
What should I know before I start insulin? 77
Should I give insulin before the meal or after the meal? 78
Should I eat snacks on an insulin regimen? 78
What should I do if I have low sugar? 79
What happened when my sugar is not low, but I feel like my sugar is low? 79
What is happening when I check my sugar and it is low, but I do not feel like it is low? 79
What can I do to recognize the hypoglycemia unawareness? 80
What bizarre behaviors do your friends and family need to pay attention to? 80
How do I regain hypoglycemia awareness? 81
Is CGM the best way to prevent hypoglycemia? 81

Chapter 9: All about insulin 82

Which type of insulin is best? 82
What is long-acting insulin? 82
What is fast-acting insulin? 82
Are there any other types of insulin? 83
Generic/Brand names for rapid-acting and short-acting insulins 84
Brand names for intermediate-acting and long-acting insulins 85
Brand names for premixed insulins 86
Who can use inhaled insulin? 86
What should I do if I forget long-acting insulin? 87
What should I do if I accidentally inject fast-acting insulin for long-acting insulin? 88

What should I do if I accidentally inject long-acting insulin for fast-acting insulin? 88

What should I do if I accidentally inject myself with long-acting as short-acting and short-acting as long-acting? 89

Why is pre-mixed insulin not optimal for type 1 diabetes? 90

Why are some insulins clear and other insulins cloudy? 91

How should I store insulin? 91

I do not have a good memory. I think I gave myself a shot a minute ago, but I am not sure if I did or did not. Is there anything I can do? 92

Which one is better? Pen or vial? 92

Which needle is better? 92

Where can I inject? 93

What else do I need to remember when I do an injection? 93

If I have type 2 diabetes. What can I do to prevent weight gain with insulin use? 93

Do you have general tips on how to use insulin? 94

Can you tell me more about basal and bolus regimen? 96

What is a sliding scale? How do I use it? 96

I have type 1 diabetes. Do you have general recommendations about how to adjust long-acting insulin? 96

I have type 2 diabetes. Do you have a general recommendation about how to adjust long-acting insulin? 97

Is there an app to help me to calculate my insulin dosage? 97

What should I do with those needles and sharps? 98

Chapter 10: Let's talk more about eating 99

What can I eat? 99

Can I eat fruit? Which ones are the best? 99

What are the best vegetables for diabetes? 101

I have heard that green tea is good for me. Can drinking green tea help reduce my hunger? When should I drink it? 102
What are your favorite foods, and how do you prepare them? 102
What are your recommendations for breakfast? 105
What are some of your ideas about snacks? 106
What are your first-tier snacks? 106
What are your second-tier snacks? 106
What are your third-tier snacks? 107
What is the best dressing I can use? 107
Salad dressing list 108
When is the best time to eat fruit? 111
What can I eat if my doctor does not recommend fruit for me? 111
Can I eat sugar-free cookies? 112
Can I eat sugar-free ice cream? 112
How many carbohydrates may I eat? 112
Should I calculate my calories every day? 112
What is the best diet? 113
People say fiber is good for diabetes. How much fiber should I consume every day? 113
What is a low-fat diet? Is it good for diabetes? 113
What is the DASH diet? Is it good for diabetes? 113
What is the Mediterranean diet? Is it good for diabetes? 114
Are there any other diets I can follow? 114
My potassium is low. What food is good for me? 114

Chapter 11: Let's talk about sweeteners 115

What are the Sweeteners? 115
Is Aspartame marketed as NutraSweet toxic? 116
What do we know about sucralose? 116
What is neotame? 116

What is acesulfame potassium? 117
What is saccharin? 117
What is Equal? 117
What is stevia? 117
Can I eat honey or use honey as sweetener? 118

Chapter 12: Let's answer questions about holiday eating 119

Why do holidays always mess up my diabetes control? 119
How can I lower my stress during the holidays? 120
I am short of money for the holidays. Do you have any suggestions? .. 120
Holidays have so many parties and so much food. I cannot resist all the good food and it is only once a year. What can I do? 122
I have type 1 diabetes and I am using an insulin pump. What can I do to control my holiday meals better? 122
I am taking multiple daily injections of insulin to control my diabetes. What can I do for holiday eating? 123
I am using the basal insulin. What can I do for holiday eating? 124
I am taking oral medications. Is there anything I can I do holiday eating? 124

Chapter 13: Diabetes and exercise 125

For a normal person, what does short-term exercise do to our body sugar? 125
For a normal person, what does long-term exercise do to the body? 125
Why is exercise important to diabetes? 125
I have type 2 diabetes, and otherwise I am healthy and fit. Is there anything I need to do before I exercise? 126
Can I drink Gatorade or another sport drink while I am exercising? 126
Is the G2 version better than regular Gatorade? 126
Do you recommend other sport drinks? 127
I am using a wristband to monitor my activities. Is it accurate? 128

Should I join a gym?... 128
I am too busy to do any exercise. What can I do? 128
When is it better to exercise, before a meal or after a meal?.................. 128
Is it better to exercise after a meal so I will not have hypoglycemia?... 129
I do not have time during the day. Can I do my exercise at night? 129
What kind of exercise is good for diabetes? 129
What is aerobic exercise? 129
What is resistance training? 130
I have a history of cardiovascular disease. What should I pay more attention to while exercising? 130
I have retinopathy. What should I pay more attention to while I exercise? 131
I have neuropathy. What should I remember when I do my exercise? 131
I have Charcot foot. What can I do for exercise? 131
I have nephropathy. What should I pay attention to during exercise?. 132
How should I work with a personal trainer? 132

Chapter 14: Diabetes and travel 134

Why should I have a travel plan for my diabetes?................................... 134
What and how should I prepare for my travel? 134
I have type 1 diabetes and I am using an insulin pump, how should I prepare for travel? Do you have a checklist?... 134
I have type 1 diabetes and I am on basal and bolus regimen. How should I prepare for travel? Do you have a checklist? 135
I have type 2 diabetes and I am taking insulin. What should I do to prepare for travel?.. 136
I am traveling by plane. Any TSA tips?... 136
I have type 1 diabetes, and I am on an insulin pump. I will fly over a few time zones. How do I change my pump settings? 136

I am on long-acting and short-acting insulin. I will fly east over a few time zones. What should I do?......137

I am on long-acting and short-acting insulin. I will fly west over a few time zones. What should I do to my basal insulin?......138

I am on oral diabetes medications. What should I do if I travel over a few time zones?......138

Chapter 15: How should I prepare for a colonoscopy or outpatient surgery?......140

What should I do when I am preparing for a colonoscopy?......140

What should I do if I am going to have surgery tomorrow?......142

Chapter 16: 10 questions about vaccinations......144

Why should I get vaccinated?......144

When should I get a pneumonia shot?......144

What forms of pneumonia shots do we have?......144

What pneumonia shot should I get?......144

How often should I get an influenza (flu) shot?......144

Should I get a stronger flu shot?......144

Why should I get Hepatitis B shot?......145

How often should I get Hepatitis B vaccine?......145

When should I get shingles vaccine?......145

Should I get Tdap vaccine also?......145

Chapter 17: Let's talk more about insulin pump failure.......146

Why do I need to be prepared for insulin pump failure?......146

How should I be prepared for an insulin pump failure?......146

What to do if I think my pump fails?......146

How should I take care of my insertion site?......148

My sugar is high and I have ketones. What should I do?......148

My sugar is high but I do not have high ketones. What should I do?...149

What are the most common causes for high sugar experienced by your insulin pump patients? 150

Chapter 18: Diabetes and cholesterol 151

What are lipids? 151
Why is it important to control lipids in diabetes? 151
What items are in the routine lipid profile test? 151
What kind of lipid profile do we see in diabetes patients? 152
Why do the triglyceride numbers change a lot from tests at different times? 152
Do we have a target to control our lipids? 152
Do I need to have a fasting lab test or not? 153
I have a history of statin intolerance. Can I use statins again? ... 153
What do you recommend for statin intolerant patients? 153
What are other potential side effects of statins? 154
Do statins really cause diabetes or make diabetes worse? 154
Why do statins cause diabetes? 155
Should I stop statins? 155
Is there anything I can do to reduce the effect of statins on my diabetes? 155
Is it useful to take Coenzyme Q10 to alleviate the side effects of statins? 155
I have diabetes and renal failure. Should I be on statins? 156
I have diabetes and renal failure. Which statins should I use? .. 156
I am on hemodialysis. Should I stay on statins? 156
I have a renal transplant. Do you have any recommendations? ... 157
Should I use Zetia? 157
What age should I start cholesterol treatment? 157
I want to know my cardiovascular risk. Do you know any tools I can use to calculate my risk? 158

I have a renal transplant and I am on cyclosporine. What is the recommendation for statin choices? 158

I have a renal transplant and I am not taking cyclosporine. Do I have to restrict the dose of statins? 159

When do we use the new cholesterol-lowering medications like PCSK-9 inhibitors? 159

Chapter 19: Diabetes and gastroparesis..161

My doctor said I have diabetic gastroparesis. What is it? 161

Does diabetes sometimes cause gastroparesis?..161

How common is diabetic gastroparesis? 161

How is gastroparesis diagnosed?..161

Is there anything I need to know before my doctor gives me a diagnosis of gastroparesis?..162

Which medications can slow down gastric emptying? 162

Are there any medications other than diabetes medications that can delay gastric emptying?...163

Are there any other medical conditions that can mimic gastroparesis? 163

Is there anything can I do to mitigate the symptoms?............................164

Do I need to take extra vitamins for gastroparesis?................................165

My doctor put me on a medication called metoclopramide. When I read the side effects, they are very severe. Should I continue taking it?..165

Domperidone was recommended to me, but it is not FDA approved in the US. Where can I buy it? 165

How can macrolide antibiotics help relieve gastroparesis? 166

Can I take macrolide antibiotics long term?..166

What are the risks of using macrolide antibiotics? 166

Why is cisapride not readily available in US?...166

Why does my sugar vary widely from very low to very high? 166

What can we do about my unstable sugar?...167

Chapter 20: Diabetic foot care 168

Why should I check my feet every day? 168
I cannot see the bottom of my feet. What can I do? 168
What daily foot care should I do? 168
Why are my feet very dry and cracked? 168
What brand is the best cream or moisturizer for diabetic dry feet? 168
What should I do if I find a small cut or scratches on my foot? 168
What should I do if I have a deep cut? 169
When should I get a tetanus shot? 169
What is the most important thing to do to prevent future cuts? 169
When should I see a doctor for a cut? 169
I have a blister on my foot. What should I do? 169
I have calluses. What should I do? 170
I just found an ulcer on my foot. What should I do? 170
No matter what I do, I have freezing cold feet. Is there anything you can suggest? 171
I have found that I have a black toe. What should I do? 171
I have diabetic neuropathy and I have burning pain in my feet. It is so bad that I cannot sleep. What should I do? 172

Chapter 21: Diabetes and sexual dysfunction 173

How common is the problem of sexual dysfunction in men with diabetes? 173
Why do men with diabetes have erectile dysfunction? 173
I am over 60, why should I care about sex? 173
I am embarrassed. How should I raise this issue with my doctor? 174
What can I do to prevent ED? 174
Should I stop drinking? 174
What should I do if I have ED? 174

Is there anything else I can do if my insurance does not pay for Viagra, Levitra, Stendra, or Cialis? 175
Can I buy ED drugs online? 175
Are there any herbs I can try? 176
What do I need to know before I try prescription medications like Viagra, Levitra, Stendra, and Cialis? 176
Is there anything I can do about my performance anxiety? 176
Should I have my doctor check my testosterone? 177
When should I check my testosterone? 177
My testosterone was at a low level. Should I get it treated? 177

Chapter 22: Living with someone who has diabetes 178

What are the challenges in families with someone who has diabetes? .178
How can I help my spouse to understand the disease? 178
My spouse is always nagging me about my diabetes. What can I do?..178
When should I listen to my spouse? 179
My spouse is like the "diabetes police," I feel like a criminal who is under surveillance 24 hours a day. I hate this. What can I do?..............179
I lost my libido. What should I do? 180
I still have libido, but I have ED. What can I do? 180
Since my diagnosis of diabetes, my spouse prepares salads for every meal. I feel like a rabbit. I hate the food. What can I do? 181
My spouse now prepares two sets of meals, one for me, which is very bland, and one for everyone else, which is all the food I like. I cannot resist eating their food. What can I do? 181
I am feeling that I am dragging my spouse and whole family down. I am depressed. What should I do? 182

Chapter 23: Questions about diabetes emergencies 183

What is diabetic ketoacidosis? 183
What is the mortality rate for DKA? 183

What other damage might DKA do to your body? 184
What causes diabetic ketoacidosis? 184
What are the symptoms of diabetic ketoacidosis? 185
Should I see a doctor? 185
Is there anything I can do to prevent diabetic ketoacidosis? 185
How is diabetic ketoacidosis treated? 186
What is a hyperosmolar hyperglycemic state (HHS)? 186
What are the symptoms of a hyperosmolar hyperglycemic state? 187
What are the factors which can cause a hyperosmolar hyperglycemic state? 187
Is there a test for a hyperosmolar hyperglycemic state? 187
What can I do to prevent a hyperosmolar hyperglycemic state? 188
How is a hyperosmolar hyperglycemic state treated? 189

Final Words 190

What are your final words on diabetes? 190

Made in the USA
Lexington, KY
25 June 2017